HEALTHY GOURMET INDIAN COOKING

By

Arvinda Chauhan
Preena Chauhan

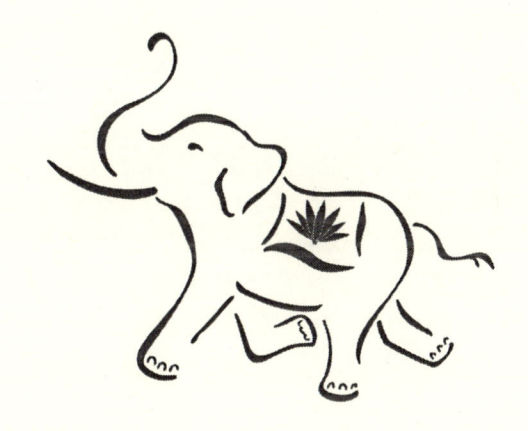

HEALTHY GOURMET INDIAN COOKING

A simple & healthy approach to Indian cuisine

Arvinda Chauhan
Preena Chauhan

AuthorHouse™
1663 Liberty Drive, Suite 200
Bloomington, IN 47403
www.authorhouse.com
Phone: 1-800-839-8640

© 2009 Arvinda Chauhan. All rights reserved.

No part of this book may be reproduced, stored in a retrieval system, or transmitted by any means without the written permission of the author.

First published by AuthorHouse 08/12/09

ISBN: 978-1-4033-3935-5 (sc)
ISBN: 978-1-4033-3936-2 (hc)
ISBN: 978-1-4033-3934-8 (e)

Printed in the United States of America
Bloomington, Indiana

ACKNOWLEDGEMENTS

I would like to thank those who cannot be forgotten, especially my grandfather whom I gratefully cooked for at an early age when I was taking care of him and my siblings. He has given me everlasting wisdom and courage. Thank you to my father for his continuous support, and for encouraging me to always strive harder and further. He always said if I let my creativity go, I could be an entrepreneur like him.

Lastly, I would like to acknowledge the many students I've taught over the years, my culinary colleagues and my family. Thank you for the continuous support, kind words and encouragement – without it my culinary experience would not be the same.

~ Arvinda Chauhan

CONTENTS

ACKNOWLEDGEMENTS v
FORWARD ix

PART 1: INGREDIENTS MATTER 1

INDIAN KITCHEN ESSENTIALS 3
- THE INDIAN SPICE BOX 5
- THE INDIAN KITCHEN 9

PREPARE INDIAN MILK PRODUCTS AT HOME 11
- PANEER 12
- GHEE 13
- ORGANIC HOMEMADE YOGURT 14

PART 2: COOKING WITH ARVINDA'S RECIPES 17

APPETIZERS, STARTERS & SNACKS 19
- ALOO WADAS 20
- DAL WADAS 22
- WHOLE VEGETABLE PAKORAS 24
- MIXED VEGETABLE PAKORAS 26
- CURRIED PUMPKIN APPLE SOUP 28
- TIKKA POTATOES 30
- SEASONED TOFU 32
- CURRIED MAPLED WALNUTS 33

CHUTNEY, RAITA & SALAD 35
- CURRIED APPLE PRESERVES 36
- MADRAS VEGETABLE RAITA 37
- CARROT & CABBAGE SAMBAR 38

FLATBREADS 41
- METHI THEPLA 42
- MASALA PURI 44

INDIAN BRUNCH 47
- GARAM MASALA OMELETTES 48
- INDIAN-STYLE PANCAKES 49
- MADRASI FRENCH TOAST 50
- CHAI VANILLA YOGURT with SEASONAL SOFT FRUIT & WALNUTS 51

VEGETARIAN CURRIES 53
- ALOO GOBI 54
- MIXED VEGETABLE CURRY 56
- SPICED POTATO & EGGPLANT CURRY 58
- MATTAR PANEER 60

LENTILS & BEANS 63
- BLACK-EYED BEAN CURRY with SPINACH 64
- CHANNA DAL with ZUCCHINI 66
- MASOOR DAL 68
- CURRIED CARROT MASOOR DAL SOUP with WHIPPED YOGURT 70
- SPROUTED MOONG BEANS 72
- CHANNA MASALA 74

NON-VEGETARIAN CURRIES 77
- CLASSIC CHICKEN CURRY 78
- CURRIED FISH 80
- MASALA CHOPS 82
- MADRAS CURRY 84
- BOILED EGG CURRY 86
- SHEIKH KEBABS with VEGETABLES 88
- CHICKEN TIKKA 90
- TANDOORI CHICKEN 92

RICE 95
- VEGETABLE JEWELLED PULLAO 96
- CURRIED RICE 98

DESSERTS & SWEET BEVERAGES 101
- MASALA CHAI 102
- CHAI VANILLA ICE CREAM with COCONUT & CRANBERRIES 104
- CRUNCHY CHAI ALMOND CHOCOLATE & CHERRY BISCOTTI 105
- CHAI GINGER RHUBARB APPLES with SEASONAL BERRY COMPOTE 106

PART 3: HEALTHY GOURMET INDIAN COOKING RECIPES 109
- ALOO WADAS 110
- MIXED VEGETABLE PAKORAS 112
- GREEN CILANTRO & MINT CHUTNEY 114
- SWEET & SOUR TAMARIND DATE CHUTNEY 116
- SWEET APPLE CHUTNEY 117
- MANGO PICKLES 118
- COOL CUCUMBER RAITA 119

KACHUMBER	120
CARROT & CABBAGE SAMBAR	122
CHAPPATI	124
PURI	126
ALOO GOBI	128
CHANNA DAL WITH ZUCCHINI	130
MASOOR DAL	132
CHANNA MASALA	134
BOILED OR STEAMED RICE	136
JEERA RICE	137
MATTAR RICE	138
INDIAN-STYLE RICE PUDDING WITH SAFFRON & NUTS	140
MANGO LASSI	142
GAJJAR KA HALWA	143

APPENDICES ..... A
   Table of Conversions ..... B
   Arvinda's Artisanal Spice Blends C

INDEX

FORWARD

I started cooking Indian food at a very early age, basically out of necessity when my mother passed away. I experienced grinding fresh flour through a heavy grinding stone and pounding spices in a large mortar and pestle, while cooking for my siblings before and after school. My very first cooking experience was making chappatis on a *chula*, a coal heated clay stove, a practice still carried out in rural parts of India today. It was my childhood experience that helped me develop my extensive knowledge of Indian cuisine over many years.

What initially started out as an obligation, cooking later turned into a passion as my creative energies became expressed through food. I started experimenting with both regional Indian cooking styles and world cuisine in my kitchen as it was something I really loved to do, and later realized I was itching to share my knowledge with others. In 1993, at a time when Indian cuisine was just getting popular in North America, I started Healthy Gourmet Indian Cooking school (www.hgic.ca).

Our cooking classes feature healthy, home-style classic recipes designed for everyday Indian cooking. Our students are delighted that after taking only a few cooking classes they gain the confidence to cook up a storm of delicious Indian dishes with the knowledge of using the right combination of spices and a few key ingredients.

The recipes in this cookbook feature wholesome, delicious and home-style recipes to be enjoyed everyday. Many of the recipes suggest variations so feel free to tailor your dishes to your liking. We promote using local and seasonal produce, so make substitutions where you see fit to eat in accordance with what is available in the markets (e.g. use sun-ripened organic tomatoes when in season in lieu of canned crushed or ground tomatoes). Just keep in mind you may get slightly different results.

Since this book features recipes for everyday cooking, we understand the reality of blending, grinding and roasting spices—an integral part of Indian cooking—is not always quick, easy and economical using numerous individual spices. Therefore we added a special section called "Cooking with Arvinda's", which substitute individual spices with Arvinda's artisanal spice blends for Indian cooking (www.arvindas.com). When we started teaching in the early 90s, we understood our time-pressed students needed to learn how to whip up great Indian meals quickly or with fewer steps, without having to compromise authenticity and taste. We developed a number of masalas (mixtures of spices) derived from family recipes and sold them through our cooking classes. The students absolutely loved them as it helped them make complex dishes more easily and conveniently. With raving reviews, my son Paresh and daughter Preena thought it would be great to someday bring them to market.

While doing her Masters degree in Environmental Studies in 2005, Preena had the opportunity to start her own company. Naturally, it was the masalas and spice blends sold through the cooking school that immediately came to mind. Shortly thereafter, Arvinda's line of artisanal spice blends for Indian cooking was born. Today, Arvinda's is sold in gourmet, specialty retailers and health food stores. For recipes and more information visit www.arvindas.com.

The "Cooking with Arvinda's" section contains easy, mouth-watering recipes using our signature spice blends for your convenience. Please keep in mind Arvinda's blends are very concentrated and a little goes a long way. In this section all the recipes will make dishes with a medium heat, so if you prefer milder flavours reduce the amount of masala called for in the recipe (e.g. reduce 1 tbsp to 2 tsp for a milder, subtle version). For more heat, add 1 tsp extra. Even in our home where fresh meals are prepared everyday, we're dependent on Arvinda's spice blends for versatility, time saving and convenience—whether we're cooking for two people or a crowd of twenty. We hope you love them too!

For your reference, many of the same recipes can also be found in the last section—"Healthy Gourmet Indian Cooking recipes" using individual spices. All our recipes use wholesome, unprocessed and natural ingredients showing you the real essence of authentic Indian cooking, each serving 2-4 people unless otherwise stated.

We welcome you to our kitchen and our world of Indian cooking and hoping you will join us for a cooking class or two!

PART 1

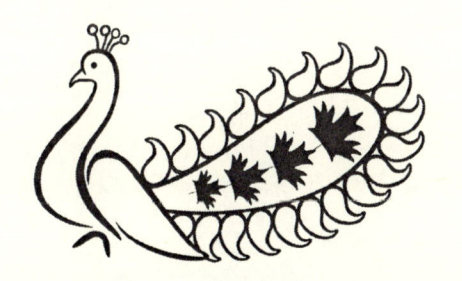

INGREDIENTS MATTER

Spices, Ingredients & Utensils

Arvinda and Preena Chauhan

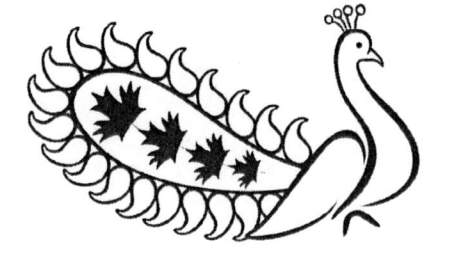

INDIAN KITCHEN ESSENTIALS

The quality of your ingredients can 'make or break' the outcome of your curry, so it is essential your ingredients are chosen with the utmost care. Freshness both in produce and spices will contribute to a superior quality curry. To ensure your spices are of the highest quality, purchase them in small quantities so unused spices are not wasting away in your pantry. Spices and dried herbs lose their flavour and aroma after nine months to a year. Store them in airtight containers or jars in a cool, dark place in your kitchen to extend their shelf life. Favouring local, seasonal and organic produce wherever possible will also amplify the flavour and taste in all your Indian curries and dishes.

Arvinda and Preena Chauhan

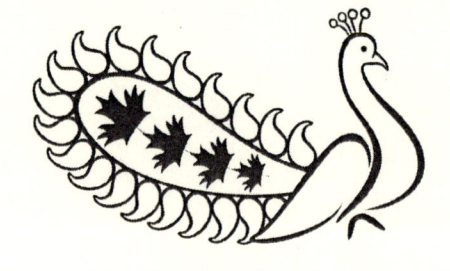

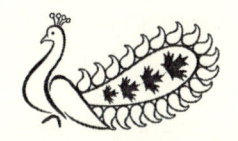

THE INDIAN SPICE BOX

Listed below are spices and ingredients most commonly used in Indian cuisine.

Ajwan seeds: Strongly flavoured, bitter and pungent, ajwan seeds are tiny grayish-brown seeds used in Indian vegetarian dishes, snacks and flatbreads. Sometimes referred to as bishop's weed.

Asafoetida: Known as *hing*, this spice has a pungent odour and is bitter to taste, therefore is always used in a very small quantity. Usually a pinch is all you need in most dishes. It is often used in vegetable, bean and lentil dishes to aid in digestion. Its flavour is reminiscent in savoury pappadums and spicy pickles.

Cardamom: Native to the rainforests of South India, green cardamom pods contain tiny black fragrant seeds, imparting an intensely strong flavour to Indian dishes. Green cardamom pods known for their sweeter quality are versatile and can be used whole or ground in both sweet and savoury dishes including rice pullao, curries and Indian desserts.

Chick pea flour: Also known as gram flour or *besan*, this flour is derived from channa dal lentils and is used as a thickener for curry sauces, and in batters for Indian flatbreads, desserts and snacks such as Pakoras or Bhajias.

Chilies: The fruit of capsicum plant and native to tropical America, chilies were introduced to India by the Portuguese. Chili powder is one of the most important spices used in Indian cuisine, as it is the ingredient that renders a fiery hotness to a dish. Add according to your taste.

Cinnamon: Native to Sri Lanka, cinnamon comes from the fragrant bark of the laurel tree and has a rich, sweet flavour. Add whole sticks to meat dishes, sweet chutneys and rice dishes.

Cloves: Native to the Moluccan Islands of Indonesia and grown in India for over a century, cloves are used whole in curries and rice dishes or may be fried, roasted or ground according to the recipe. Cloves are known for its medicinal value of acting as a mild anesthetic hence it is commonly used to relieve toothaches. Also an anti-bacterial agent, a steaming cup of Masala Chai containing aromatic cloves is known to soothe a sore throat.

Coriander seeds: The round seeds of the coriander plant are an essential spice to almost all Indian dishes, imparting a mellow, citrusy flavour to an Indian dish. It is most often used ground before use. Fresh coriander leaves (also known as cilantro or Chinese parsley) is a widely available, aromatic herb used in fresh chutneys and sauces and as a garnish on top of curries and rice dishes.

Cumin seeds: Known as *jeera*, cumin seeds are used either whole or ground into a powder. Aiding in digestion, cumin is one of the most frequently used spice in Indian curries and rice dishes. Whole seeds are roasted and ground for use in raita, salads and chutneys.

Curry leaves: An important herb in South Indian cooking, this dark green leaf has a distinctive, citrusy and tangy flavour. It pairs nicely with potato, vegetable and lentil dishes, and is an important ingredient in the Goan dish, Vindaloo.

Dal: Beans or pulses which are split and/or hulled, is known as dal. Dal also refers to a specific dish of soupy, spicy lentil soup.

Fennel seeds: These small greenish seeds with a licorice-like flavour have been used for centuries in both cooking and for medicinal purposes. Commonly served at the end of an Indian meal, fennel acts as a natural breath sweetener and counteracts nausea, bloating, gas and indigestion.

Fenugreek seeds: The yellow seeds of the fenugreek plant are highly aromatic and strongly flavoured and are commonly used in meat dishes and pickles. Fenugreek leaves, known as *methi* are used in flatbreads, Indian snacks and vegetable dishes.

Garam masala: This quintessential Indian pantry staple is a blend of aromatic spices including cinnamon, cardamom, nutmeg and peppercorns, adding warmth to an Indian curry or rice pullao. Sprinkle Garam Masala as a garnish on top of any dish as the final layer of spicing – most curries are incomplete without it!

Garlic: Used widely in Indian cuisine, garlic is usually in the form of garlic puree or paste (pure garlic without salt or oil).

Ghee (clarified butter): Ghee is regular butter that has the milk solids and salts removed from it. To make your own ghee at home, follow our easy and simple recipe in the book. Ghee is a quintessential ingredient in rice dishes and desserts.

Ginger: Used widely in Indian cooking primarily in the form of a paste or a puree (pure ginger with no added salt or oil).

Jaggery: Derived from sugarcane jaggery is used as a wholesome and unrefined sweetening agent. In India it is known as *gur*.

Masala: A generic term meaning mixture of spices.

Mustard seeds: These dark brown little seeds are an important spice in Southern Indian, Bengali and vegetarian cooking. When placed in hot oil, mustard seeds pop and release an intense flavour.

Nutmeg: An important spice in Chai Masala and Garam Masala, nutmeg has a mild, sweet flavour and a gentle aroma ideal for Indian sweets. Purchase nutmeg whole and grate as needed.

Saffron: The most expensive spice, saffron comes from the stigmas and upper part of the styles of the crocus flower. Orange-red in color, saffron is used sparingly in festive dishes such as Biryani, meat curries desserts and drinks.

Tamarind: Sour and brown in colour, tamarind is used widely in meat, poultry and dal dishes as well as in chutneys.

Turmeric: Yellow in colour, turmeric is India's 'superspice', an antioxidant, containing an abundance of medicinal value including aiding in digestion and acting as an anti-bacterial agent. Turmeric gives curry its unique yellow colour. Use in small quantities to avoid bitterness.

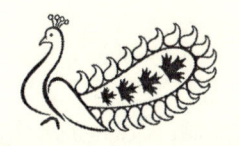

THE INDIAN KITCHEN

To cook authentic Indian meals at home requires only a handful of these basic utensils.

Belan: A thin rolling pin used for making Indian flatbreads and samosa pastries, this rolling pin allows you to make chappati into perfect circles. Extremely versatile, you can use it for your everyday baking.

Food processor: Used for processing ingredients to make fine pastes such as lentil wada mixtures, chutneys and garlic and ginger paste.

Ghee container: A small stainless steel container to store prepared ghee.

Kadhai: A large wok-like utensil for deep frying and sautéing. It can be made out of stainless steel, iron or brass.

Masala box (masala dabba): A round, stainless steel container which stores up to seven different spices. Masala boxes come in various sizes—small, medium and large and include an airtight lid helping to extend the shelf life of spices. Store your masala box in a cool, dark place.

Mortar and pestle: Used to coarsely grind spices, nuts or other ingredients.

Parat: A shallow, stainless steel dish with high edges used to knead Indian flatbread dough.

Pressure cooker: A good quality stainless steel pressure cooker is essential in an Indian kitchen to cook curries, lentils and beans. This can cut down the cooking time of beans and lentils from 1 hour to 10-15 minutes. Always follow enclosed instructions to ensure the safety of using the pressure cooker is exercised at all times.

Stainless Steel Saucepan: Heavy bottom stainless steel pan used for cooking any Indian dishes. Non-stick saucepans are ideal for making rice dishes or dry curries.

Tawa: A griddle made out of caste iron used for making Indian flatbreads on high temperature. A frying pan or skillet is a good substitute.

Thali: A stainless steel dish or tray with a variety of small bowls to serve a full Indian meal. Restaurants often serve a vegetarian thali of a variety of rice, lentil and vegetable dishes, chutneys and an Indian sweet.

PREPARE INDIAN MILK PRODUCTS at HOME

Milk, nature's nectar of life is used in so many different ways in Indian cuisine and is often the main ingredient in many recipes. Diary products are a staple all over India especially in Punjab, India's northwestern state. Using these simple recipes, you can make your own organic milk products at home.

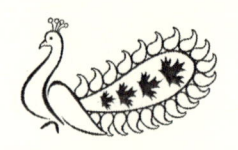

PANEER
Homemade Indian cheese

Ingredients:

4 cups	organic homogenized milk
¼ cup	vinegar or lemon juice

Method of Preparation:

Bring milk to boil. Turn off the heat.

Add vinegar or lemon juice and stir until the milk curdles and water separates.

Strain through a thin muslin or cheesecloth. Wrap the curdled milk in a cloth and flatten to form a square. Place a heavy weight over the paneer square overnight or 6-8 hours to drain out water.

Remove cloth gently and cut into cubes. Add paneer cubes to your favourite curry. Try homemade paneer in Mattar Paneer (see recipe in book).

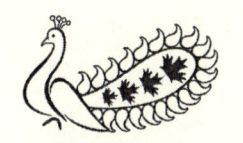

GHEE
Clarified butter

Cooking spices in ghee is advantageous as it allows for spices to be 'tempered' without burning them. Ghee has a nutty flavour and is one of Indian cuisine's quintessential ingredients used in curries, flatbreads, desserts and rice pullao. Oil can be substituted for ghee however it will lack the same beautiful flavour that ghee lends to a dish.

Ingredients:

½ lb   unsalted butter

Method of Preparation:

In a small saucepan, melt butter and cook on low heat. Continue to cook ghee until a transparent liquid is formed at the top and milk residue settles at the bottom of the pan.

Once liquid is golden colour the ghee is ready. Remove from heat immediately.

Strain into a jar or ghee container with fine sieve or strainer. Ghee will keep up to four weeks when stored in the refrigerator.

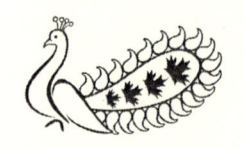

ORGANIC HOMEMADE YOGURT
Curd or 'Dhai'

Ingredients:

4 cups   organic homogenized milk
2 tbsp   plain organic yogurt

Method of Preparation:

Preheat oven to 150F degrees.

In a medium pot, bring milk to boil then turn the heat off immediately. Set milk aside until milk is lukewarm.

Transfer the milk into a medium bowl and combine with 2 tablespoons of plain organic yogurt. Whip together with a hand blender or whisk until mixture becomes frothy.

Place bowl in warm oven for 6 to 8 hours until the yogurt sets. Once the yogurt forms refrigerate immediately.

Tip:

In summer months when your kitchen temperature is higher (requires a minimum 80F/26°C), leave the bowl on the kitchen counter overnight to allow yogurt to set rather than using the oven. Energy conservation method!

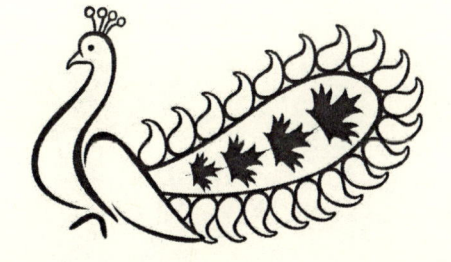

Healthy Gourmet Indian Cooking

Arvinda and Preena Chauhan

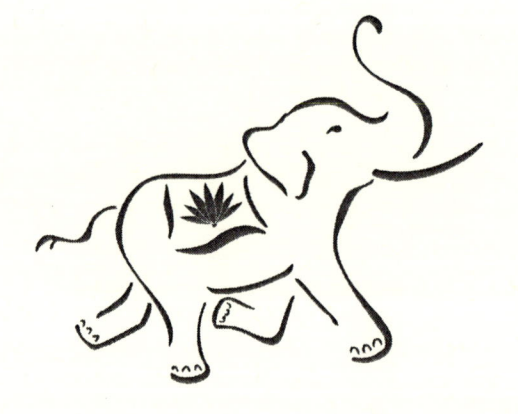

PART 2

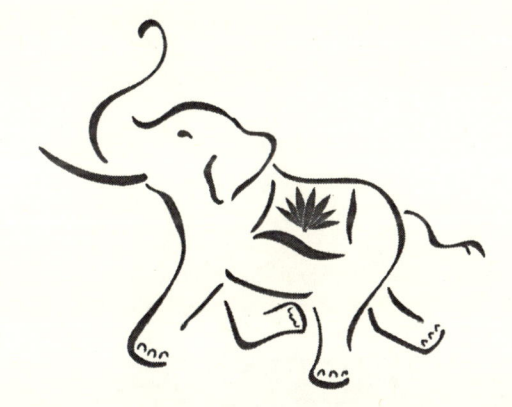

COOKING with ARVINDA's recipes

This section features recipes using Arvinda's artisanal spice blends for Indian cooking. With the help of Arvinda's, making authentic Indian classics and fusion Indian-inspired dishes has never been easier! Adjust the use of Arvinda's masalas to suit your personal palate and taste.

Arvinda and Preena Chauhan

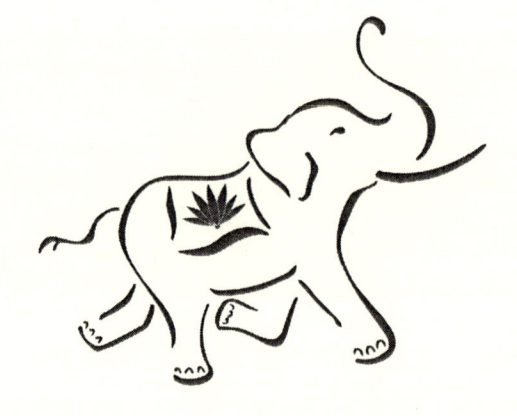

APPETIZERS, STARTERS & SNACKS

Appetizers and snacks are an important part of Indian tradition as it brings family and friends together during festivals and colourful celebrations. When one visits an Indian home, guests are naturally welcomed with a steamy hot plate of Vegetable Pakoras or any other appetizer, served with a steaming cup of Masala Chai—an expression of the true spirit of Indian hospitality.

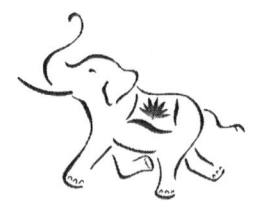

Arvinda's

ALOO WADAS
Potato & Cilantro Balls in a Crispy Chick Pea Batter

Serve this delicious starter with Green Coriander & Mint Chutney. Use Arvinda's Curry Masala in combination with Arvinda's Tikka Masala to make these Aloo Wadas especially flavourful.

Ingredients:

Batter

2 cups	chick pea flour
1 tsp	**Arvinda's Curry Masala**
¼ tsp	salt OR salt to taste
¼ tsp	baking soda
½ cup	water OR enough water to make thick batter

Filling

5	large potatoes, peeled, boiled, drained and mashed
2 tbsp	cilantro, finely chopped
2 tbsp	raisins
½ tsp	fresh lemon juice
½ tsp	salt OR salt to taste
1 tsp	**Arvinda's Tikka Masala**
½ tsp	**Arvinda's Garam Masala**
	oil for deep frying

Method of Preparation:

Batter: In a medium bowl sift chick pea flour.

Add **Arvinda's Curry Masala,** salt and baking powder. Add enough water to make a thick, smooth batter. If the batter is too thin, add extra sifted chick pea flour to thicken it up. Batter should be a thick consistency. Set aside to rest.

Filling: In a large bowl, mix mashed potatoes with the rest of the filling ingredients. Mix well and set aside to cool.

Take a small lump of the filling mixture the size of a walnut and form a smooth ball. Continue to mold the remaining mixture the same way.

In a kadhai or wok, heat oil for deep-frying on medium heat.

Dip potato balls in chick pea flour batter, coating well. Slide each ball into the oil carefully. Fry until golden brown. Remove from oil and drain on a paper towel.

Tip:
Aloo wadas can be prepared and fried ahead of time and reheated in the oven just before serving.

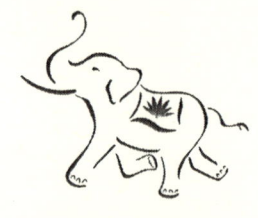

Arvinda's

DAL WADAS
Lentil Fritters

These appetizers can be served with any Indian chutney or can be served as a light lunch (similar to falafel) in a pita pocket with chopped lettuce, tomatoes and cucumber, topped off with Raita, a yogurt condiment.

Ingredients:

1 cup	moong dal, washed
1	small onion, peeled and finely chopped
2 tbsp	cilantro, finely chopped
2 tsp	**Arvinda's Curry Masala**
1 tsp	sesame seeds
½ tsp	salt OR salt to taste
¼ tsp	baking soda
	oil for deep frying

Method of Preparation:

Wash moong dal in several changes of warm water. Soak and set aside for one hour.

Drain moong dal. In a food processor, grind drained moong dal into a course thick paste.

Transfer into a mixing bowl and add chopped onion, cilantro, **Arvinda's Curry Masala**, sesame seeds, salt and baking soda. Mix well and set aside for 5 minutes.

In a kadhai or wok, heat oil for deep-frying on medium heat.

Mold mixture into small balls. Fry a few wadas at a time, and cook for 3-4 minutes until golden brown.

Serve hot or cold with Indian chutneys.

Tip:
When deep frying always drain on a paper towel to absorb excess oil.

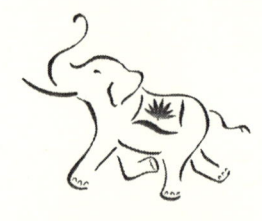

Arvinda's

WHOLE VEGETABLE PAKORAS
Whole Vegetable Fritters in a Chick Pea Flour Batter

This is the recipe to try, the next time you want to impress your guests with something delicious. It's easy too!

Ingredients:

Batter mixture

2 cups	chick pea flour
1 tsp	**Arvinda's Curry Masala**
½ tsp	salt OR salt to taste
¼ tsp	baking powder OR baking soda
¾ cup	water to make batter

Vegetables

4	cauliflower OR broccoli florets, separated into smaller pieces
1	small potato, peeled and sliced into rounds
1	small zucchini, cut into thin slices
1	small onion, sliced
1	green pepper, seeded and sliced into rings
2 cups	light cooking oil for deep frying

Method of Preparation:

Batter: In a mixing bowl, combine chick pea flour, **Arvinda's Curry Masala**, salt and baking soda. Add water to make a thick batter. Mix well and let stand for 5 minutes.

In a kadhai or wok, heat oil for deep-frying on medium heat.

Dip vegetables one by one into the batter, coat well and fry for a few minutes until golden brown. Turn vegetables to fry on both sides.

Drain well on a paper towel. Serve hot or cold with chutney.

Tip:

Try making these Pakoras with pineapple rings, green chilies, semi ripe bananas, boneless chicken cubes or fish pieces for a variation.

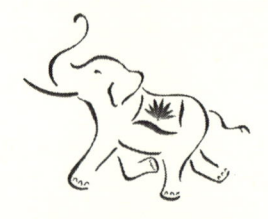

Arvinda's

MIXED VEGETABLE PAKORAS
Mixed Vegetable Chick Pea Fritters

Ingredients:

Batter mixture

2 cup	chick pea (besan OR gram) flour
2 tsp	**Arvinda's Curry Masala**
1 tsp	salt OR salt to taste
¼ tsp	baking powder OR baking soda
1 tbsp.	water

Vegetables

2	small potatoes, peeled, finely chopped
1	small zucchini, finely chopped
1	small onion, finely chopped
1	green pepper, seeded, finely chopped
1	small ripe banana, finely chopped (optional)
¼ cup	cilantro OR spinach, finely chopped
2 cup	light cooking oil for deep frying

Method of Preparation:

Batter: In a mixing bowl, combine chick pea flour, **Arvinda's Curry Masala**, salt and baking soda. Add water, mix and combine to make a thick batter.

Add chopped vegetables. Mix well and allow to stand for 5 minutes.

In a kadhai or wok, heat oil for deep-frying on medium heat.

Take a teaspoon of pakora mixture and carefully drop into oil. Fry a few at a time. Fry on all sides until golden brown.

Drain well on a paper towel. Serve hot or cold with chutneys.

Tip:

This appetizer is a good option for anyone who has a gluten allergy as it contains no wheat. If you don't have a spicy chutney on hand, serve these pakoras with ketchup.

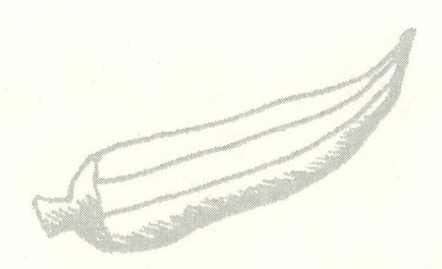

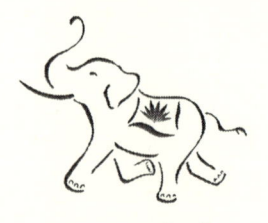

Arvinda's

CURRIED PUMPKIN APPLE SOUP

This is a wonderful warm and comforting soup for the colder months using locally harvested pumpkins and apples of the fall season.

Ingredients:

¼	small pumpkin, skin removed, cut into small cubes
1	apples, cored with the skins removed and cubed
4 cups	vegetable stock
2 tsp	**Arvinda's Curry Masala** (add more to taste for a spicier soup)
½ cup	light cream
1 tsp	sugar
¼ cup	chopped cilantro, to garnish
½ tsp	**Arvinda's Garam Masala,** to garnish

Method of Preparation:

In a large pot add water, pumpkin and apples and cook on high heat for approximately 20-30 minutes or until cooked.

Puree with a hand blender until smooth.

Add vegetable stock, **Arvinda's Curry Masala** and sugar. Stir and simmer on medium heat for 10 minutes. Add light cream, sea salt to taste. Add additional **Arvinda's Curry Masala** to get soup to desired hotness.

Add additional water, if necessary to give a soupy consistency.

Serve soup in a bowl garnished with a sprinkle of **Arvinda's Garam Masala** and chopped cilantro.

Serve with a soft, fresh French baguette and a chick pea salad to make a complete healthy meal.

Arvinda's

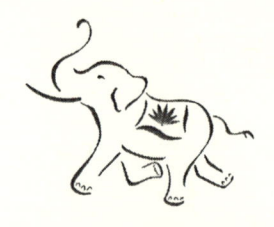

TIKKA POTATOES
Tikka Masala Pan-Fried Potatoes

Serve as a side — perfect for BBQ season!
(See photo on cover).

Ingredients:

1 lb	potatoes (5-6 medium size), peeled and cubed OR cut into wedges
1 tsp	salt
1 tbsp	oil
6-8	**Arvinda's Curry Leaves**
1 tbsp	**Arvinda's Tikka Masala** (OR use 2 tsp. for milder, subtle flavour)
1 tbsp	cilantro, coarsely chopped

Method of Preparation:

In a large pot, add water, salt and potatoes. Boil until potatoes are tender. Drain and set aside.

In a large skillet, heat oil on medium heat. Add **Arvinda's Curry Leaves** and **Arvinda's Tikka Masala**. Fry in oil for one minute.

Fold in potatoes and stir to combine thoroughly. Cook and fry over a low heat until slightly crispy.

Transfer into a serving dish and garnish with cilantro. Serve with an Indian BBQ as a side.

Tip:

Chill Tikka Potatoes and add mayonnaise, sour cream or yogurt for a cool summer potato salad with a spicy kick! Try this recipe with organic sweet potatoes for a variation.

Arvinda's

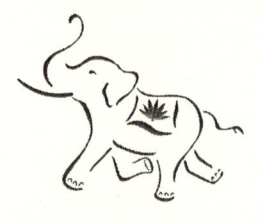

SEASONED TOFU

Season plain tofu with one of Arvinda's cooking masalas to add lots of good flavour. Extra firm tofu works best.

Ingredients:

1 pkg	extra firm organic tofu, cubed
½ cup	yogurt (optional)
1 tsp	**Arvinda's Madras, Tikka** OR **Tandoori Masala**
1 tbsp	oil

Method of Preparation:

In a medium bowl, combine yogurt, **Arvinda's Madras, Tikka** or **Tandoori Masala.** Mix well.

Add in tofu and mix to coat tofu well.

Cover bowl, refrigerate and marinate tofu for 4 hours.

In a skillet, add oil and heat on medium temperature.

Add marinated tofu and fry for several minutes until tofu becomes crispy and golden brown.

Sprinkle tofu cubes on top of a salad or add it to your favourite curry. Try it in the Quick & Easy Boiled Egg Curry recipe.

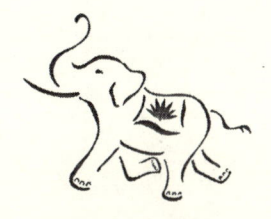

Arvinda's
CURRIED MAPLED WALNUTS

Serve these spicy nuts with drinks or sprinkle them on your favourite salads for a nice spicy bite!

Ingredients:

1¼ cup	walnut pieces
¼ cup	pure Canadian maple syrup
2 tsp	**Arvinda's Curry Masala**

Method of Preparation:

Preheat oven to 200F.

In a small bowl, combine maple syrup with **Arvinda's Curry Masala.** Mix well.

Add walnuts and coat well.

Place walnuts on a foil-lined baking sheet and bake for 5-10 minutes or until maple syrup has crystallized. Take care not to burn the nuts.

Enjoy!

Arvinda and Preena Chauhan

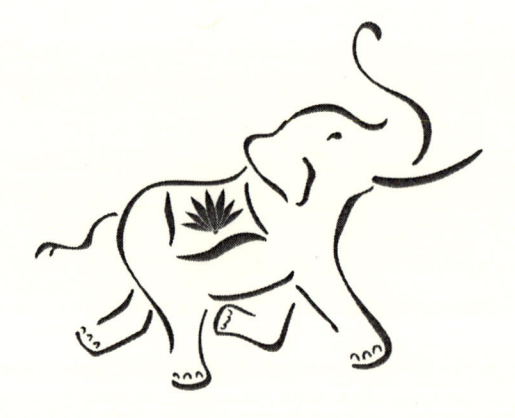

CHUTNEY, RAITA & SALAD

Alongside any complete Indian meal, a selection of chutneys, raita, and salads are present – the chutneys to add heat and extra flavour; and raita, a yogurt condiment, to cool the palate if the curries are too hot. Sweet chutneys such as apple or sweet mango compliment spicier dishes. Typical Indian salads are usually simple – a few tomatoes, radishes and onions with a light dressing of a little chili, vinegar and salt.

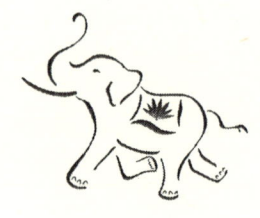

Arvinda's

CURRIED APPLE PRESERVES

Ingredients:

6	organic apples OR pears, peeled and finely cubed
¼ cup	sugar
2 tsp	**Arvinda's Curry Masala**
½ tsp	salt OR salt to taste

Method of Preparation:

In a non-stick or heavy bottom pan, combine above ingredients and cook on low heat for 45 minutes until slightly thickened. Set aside.

Once cooled, store in a glass container and refrigerate to extend shelf life.

Tip:

Serve as a condiment on a cheese plate with cheese and crackers or alongside roast turkey or pork chops.

Arvinda's

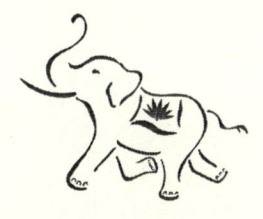

MADRAS VEGETABLE RAITA
Yogurt Condiment with Cubed Cucumber, Tomato and Spices

Ingredients:

1 cup	plain yogurt
½	English cucumber, finely cubed and drained
1	tomato, finely cubed and drained
½ tsp	**Arvinda's Madras Masala**
½ tsp	sea salt
1 tbsp	cilantro, finely chopped
pinch	**Arvinda's Garam Masala**

Method of Preparation:

In a small bowl, mix together yogurt, cucumber, tomato, **Arvinda's Madras Masala**, and salt.

Garnish with a sprinkle of cilantro and **Arvinda's Garam Masala.**

Serve chilled. This is a cool summer condiment served as a side dish.

Arvinda's

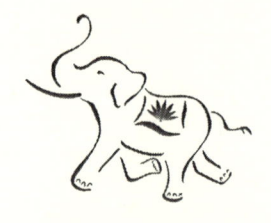

CARROT & CABBAGE SAMBAR
Sweet & Sour Warm Indian-Style Salad

Serve as a side with Indian curries, flatbread and rice.

Ingredients:

2 tsp	oil
½ tsp	brown mustard seeds
2	medium carrots, peeled and grated
1	green chilies, sliced (optional)
½	sweet red bell pepper, sliced
¼	medium cabbage, finely shredded
2 tsp	**Arvinda's Curry Masala**
1 tsp	sugar
½ tsp	salt OR salt to taste
½ tsp	lemon juice

Method of Preparation:

In a wok or kadhai, heat oil on medium high heat. Fry mustard seeds in oil until they pop.

Add carrots, chilies, bell peppers and cabbage. Combine.

Add **Arvinda's Curry Masala**, sugar, salt and lemon juice.

Mix well and stir fry for a few minutes. Be sure not to overcook vegetables. Serve as a side dish.

Tip:
Mustard seeds expand and pop when added to hot oil so cover pan with a lid when frying.

Arvinda and Preena Chauhan

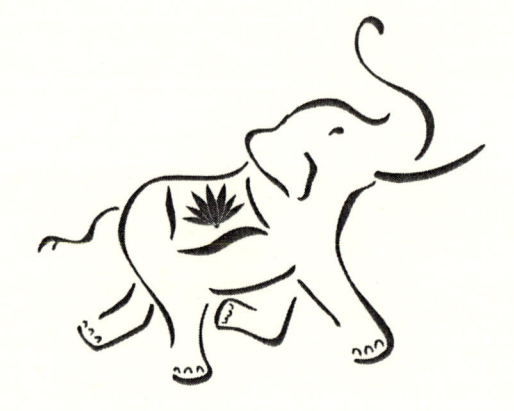

FLATBREADS

All Indian meals are accompanied with flatbreads. The flatbreads of India originate from different regions and are paired with particular dishes. For example, chappatis (round whole wheat grilled flatbread) are typically served with vegetarian dishes whereas meat dishes are served with Naan, a leavened bread. Puris, small puffed fried bread are reserved for more auspicious occasions and pair nicely with vegetarian dishes and sweets. Indian flatbreads are eaten for breakfast, lunch and dinner and are made from a variety of wholesome grains including millet, juwar (sorghum), lentil flour and rice flour. Whole wheat flour is commonly used, making Indian flatbreads both healthy and satisfying.

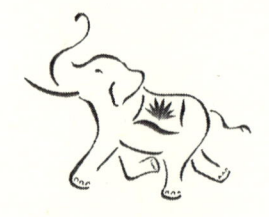

Arvinda's

METHI THEPLA
Flaky Flatbread with Spices and Fenugreek Spinach

This Indian flatbread is shallow fried and usually served at breakfast. Since this flatbread is spicy and earthy, serve it with plain yogurt.

Ingredients:

1 cup	soft whole wheat OR chappati flour
½ cup	chick pea flour
½ cup	sorgam flour (juwar) OR millet flour
2 tbsp	oil
1 tsp	sesame seeds
2 tsp	**Arvinda's Curry Masala**
1 tsp	salt
½ cup	fenugreek spinach (methi), finely chopped
½ cup	water, add more if necessary
	ghee OR oil for shallow frying

Method of Preparation:

In a large flat dish, combine all flours. Add oil, sesame seeds, **Arvinda's Curry Masala** and salt. Add chopped fenugreek spinach. Combine all the ingredients together.

Add a little water at time to make very stiff dough. Cover and set aside for 10 minutes.

Take a small lump of dough the size of a golf ball. Press between your palms to make a small patty. Roll out into a circle, relative to the size of small tortilla.

In a frying pan, cook gently on low heat on both sides until golden brown. Brush a little oil or ghee on both the sides and shallow fry them in pan.

Tip:

This flatbread will keep longer than others and can be stored up to 4 days in a tight container. It's a perfect road trip or picnic snack!

Arvinda's

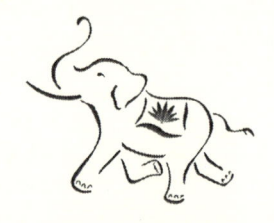

MASALA PURI
Deep-fried puris with a hint of spices

Puris are best served with Indian vegetarian curries. This recipe is a spicier variation that can be served with milder curries or with omelettes.

Ingredients:

1 cup	whole wheat flour
1 cup	duram flour OR all purpose flour
½ cup	fine semolina (suji)
2 tsp	**Arvinda's Curry Masala**
2 tsp	oil
1 tsp	sesame seeds
1 tsp	salt
½ tsp	whole cumin seeds
¾ cup	water OR enough water to make stiff dough
	oil for deep-frying

Method of Preparation:

In a large bowl, combine whole wheat flour, duram flour, semolina, **Arvinda's Curry Masala,** oil, sesame seeds, salt and cumin seeds. Mix well and knead with warm water to make stiff dough. Allow to stand covered for 5-10 minutes.

Take a small lump of dough the size of a golf ball and roll it out into a small circle on an oiled surface. Roll out three or four at a time.

In a wok, heat oil on medium heat. To test oil temperature, drop a small piece of dough in oil. When the dough surfaces immediately, the oil is ready. If not, wait for the oil to heat up further.

Slide one puri into the oil at a time. Apply gentle pressure on puri with strainer to allow puri to puff up. Turn over and allow the other side to get golden brown.

Cook for 1-2 minutes until puri becomes light golden brown on both sides.

Fry all the puris and serve hot or cold.

Serve with curries, chutneys or pickles.

Tip:

If oil fumes, the temperature is too hot. Turn down heat and resume frying when temperature is at medium high.

Arvinda and Preena Chauhan

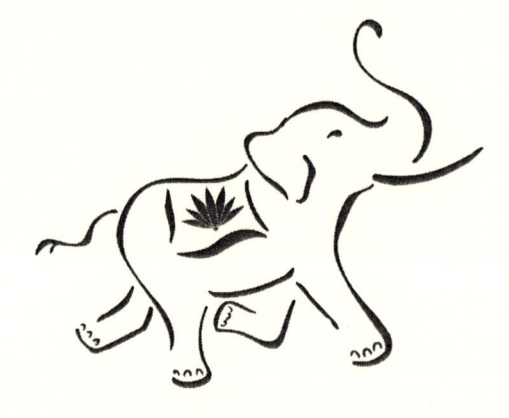

INDIAN BRUNCH

In India, many of the foods eaten for lunch or snacks such as Masala Dosas, Idli Sambhar, and Dokla (steamed savoury lentil cakes) are often served for breakfast as well. Likewise, breakfast foods can also be great for a Sunday brunch. Try these recipes for a special and spicy brunch.

Arvinda's

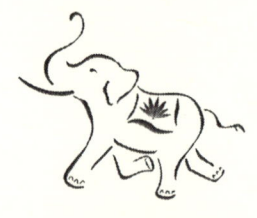

GARAM MASALA OMELETTE

Ingredients:

2	eggs
1	small onion, finely chopped
1	small tomato, finely chopped
1	green chili, finely chopped
1 tbsp	cilantro, finely chopped
¼ tsp	**Arvinda's Garam Masala**
¼ tsp	salt OR salt to taste
1 tsp	butter OR ghee

Method of Preparation:

In a small bowl, whisk eggs until frothy. Add chopped onions, tomatoes, chili, cilantro, **Arvinda's Garam Masala** and salt. Mix together.

Heat a frying pan on medium-high heat. Melt butter or ghee. Add omelette mixture and fry on both sides until slightly brown.

Serve with tomato ketchup or chutney.

Serves 1.

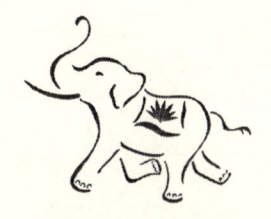

Arvinda's

INDIAN-STYLE PANCAKES

Ingredients:

½ cup	chick pea flour
2	eggs
1	medium onion, finely chopped
1 cup	spinach, finely chopped
½	zucchini, finely chopped
1 tsp	**Arvinda's Curry Masala**
½ tsp	salt
½ cup	milk
	oil for shallow frying

Method of Preparation:

In a bowl, mix together all the above ingredients (except oil). Add extra chick pea flour if necessary to make thick batter.

Heat 2 teaspoons of oil in a frying pan. Add pancake mixture to frying pan and cook on both sides until slightly brown.

Serve with raita or tomato ketchup.

Arvinda's

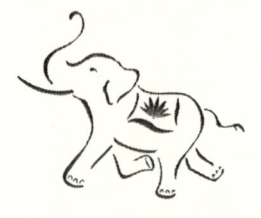

MADRASI FRENCH TOAST

Ingredients:

4 slices	whole wheat bread
2	eggs
1 tbsp	milk
1 tsp	**Arvinda's Madras Masala**
pinch	sea salt
¼ tsp	fresh ground black pepper (optional)
2 tsp	oil for shallow frying

Method of Preparation:

Toast whole wheat bread slices. Set aside.

In a small bowl, whisk together eggs, milk, **Arvinda's Madras Masala** and sea salt. Add black pepper if desired.

In a non-stick frying pan, heat a little oil on medium heat.

Transfer egg mixture in a flat dish or pie plate. Dip toasted bread into egg mixture on both sides. Place toast in frying pan. Fry on both sides until golden brown. Serve with Canadian maple syrup.

Arvinda's

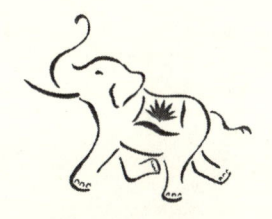

CHAI VANILLA YOGURT with SEASONAL SOFT FRUIT & WALNUTS

Ingredients:

1 cup	vanilla yogurt
1 tsp	**Arvinda's Chai Masala**
½ cup	seasonal soft fruit, chopped (raspberries, strawberries, peaches, blueberries)
1 tbsp	toasted walnuts, chopped
2 tsp	Canadian maple syrup

Method of Preparation:

In a bowl, combine vanilla yogurt and **Arvinda's Chai Masala.**

Transfer into serving bowls and garnish with seasonal fruit and chopped walnuts. Drizzle with Canadian maple syrup.

Serves 2.

Arvinda and Preena Chauhan

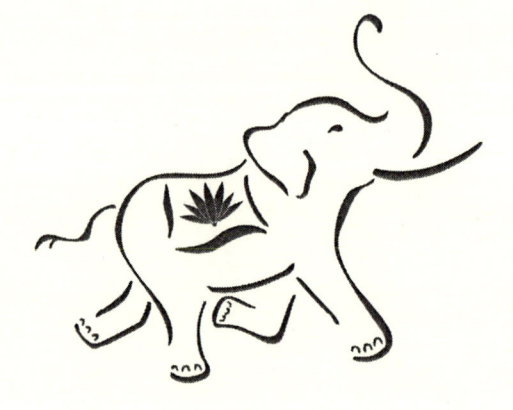

VEGETARIAN CURRIES

In Indian cuisine, an abundance of vegetables are consumed due to the fact that India is largely a country of pure vegetarians. Often vegetables are served as the main meal opposed to having vegetables as a side dish. India harvests many different varieties of vegetables—everything from bitter gourds to red carrots to okra. Try any of these recipes with local and seasonal produce. With the use of a myriad of spices, vegetables come alive.

Arvinda's

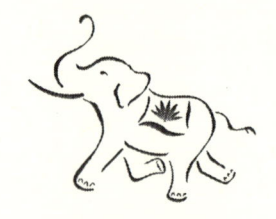

ALOO GOBI
Cauliflower and Potato Curry

This cauliflower curry is the definitive vegetarian dish. Serve with chappatis.

Ingredients:

2 tbsp	oil
½ tsp	mustard seeds
½ tsp	cumin seeds
6-8	**Arvinda's Curry Leaves**
2	medium potatoes, peeled and cubed
½	medium cauliflower, cut into small pieces
1 cup	peas
2 tbsp	**Arvinda's Curry Masala**
1 tsp	salt OR salt to taste
1 tbsp	cilantro, to garnish
½ tsp	**Arvinda's Garam Masala,** to garnish

Method of Preparation:

In a pan, heat oil on medium high temperature. Add mustard seeds and cumin seeds. Cover pan with a lid and allow to sizzle and pop. Add **Arvinda's Curry Leaves** to oil.

Add potatoes, peas and cauliflower. Reduce heat to low.

Add **Arvinda's Curry Masala** and salt. Fold in spices, coating all potatoes, peas and cauliflower.

Cover with lid and cook on low heat until potatoes are soft and cooked, approximately 20 minutes. When potatoes are cooked the dish is ready to serve.

Garnish with a sprinkle of **Arvinda's Garam Masala** and cilantro.

Tip:

Make this dish a moist curry by adding ¼ cup of canned crushed or ground tomatoes and ½ cup of water and simmer. Add ½ tsp extra of Arvinda's Curry Masala.

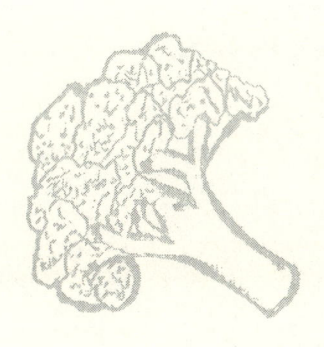

Arvinda's

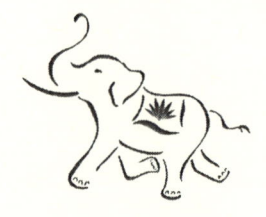

MIXED VEGETABLE CURRY

This is a delicious curry of a medley of vegetables in a tomato based sauce. Use seasonal vegetables.

Ingredients:

1 tbsp	oil
¼ tsp	black mustard seeds
¼ tsp	cumin seeds
3	medium potatoes, peeled and cubed
1	fresh tomatoes, finely chopped
1	medium eggplant, cubed
1	zucchini, cubed
½ cup	frozen green peas
1 ½ tbsp	**Arvinda's Curry Masala**
1 ½ tsp	salt OR salt to taste
½ tsp	sugar
½ tsp	tamarind paste
½ cup	water
1 tbsp	cilantro, to garnish

Method of Preparation:

In a pan, heat oil on medium heat. Fry mustard seeds and cumin seeds. Cover pot with a lid and allow to sizzle and pop for one minute.

Add potatoes, eggplants, zucchini, peas and tomatoes. Add **Arvinda's Curry Masala**, salt, sugar and tamarind paste. Mix, cover and cook for 5 minutes.

Add water, cover and cook on low heat further until potatoes and eggplants are cooked and become tender. This mixed vegetable curry should be cooked until vegetables are soft and has a thick sauce.

Garnish with cilantro. Serve with a basmati pullao.

Tip:

For this recipe, use Oriental eggplants as they will add sweetness to this dish.

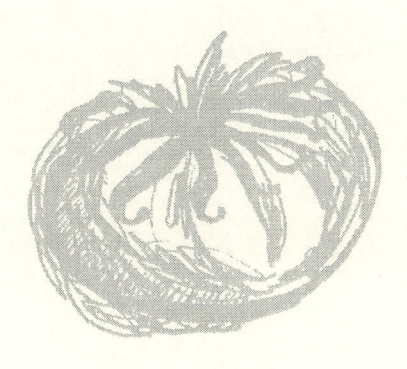

Arvinda's

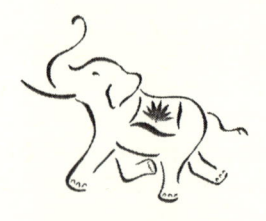

SPICED POTATO & EGGPLANT CURRY

This is a dry vegetarian dish that can be served as a side dish with dal, chappati and pickles. Serve an Indian salad and yogurt to make a complete meal.

Ingredients:

2 tbsp	oil
4-6	**Arvinda's Curry Leaves**
¼ tsp	cumin seeds
¼ tsp	mustard seeds
3	medium potatoes, peeled and thinly sliced
2	medium oriental eggplants, thinly sliced
1 ½ tbsp	**Arvinda's Curry Masala**
1 tsp	salt OR salt to taste
1 tbsp	cilantro, to garnish

Method of Preparation:

In a shallow pan, heat oil on medium high heat. Add cumin seeds and mustard seeds. Cover pot with a lid and fry until seeds pop, taking care not to burn spices. Add **Arvinda's Curry Leaves** and fry for one minute.

Add sliced potatoes and eggplant. Add **Arvinda's Curry Masala** and salt. Fold in masala to combine with potatoes and eggplant.

Cover with lid and cook on low heat until potatoes are soft for approximately 20 minutes.

Garnish with cilantro.

Tip:

Curry leaves add a citrusy burst of flavour to any vegetable dish and pair nicely with coconuts as in South Indian cooking. A simple dish of potatoes, curry leaves, sea salt and black pepper makes a wonderful side dish.

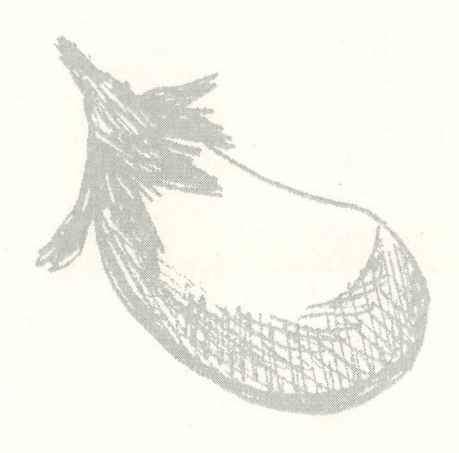

Arvinda's

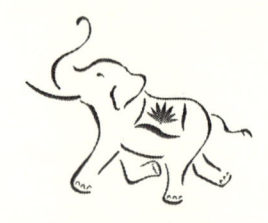

MATTAR PANEER
Indian Cheese in a Creamy Curry Sauce with Peas

Try making this dish with homemade paneer using organic milk (see homemade Paneer recipe). Paneer, sold in blocks is available at all Indian grocery stores.

Ingredients:

1 cup	paneer, cubed
1 ½ cups	frozen peas
1 tbsp	oil
3	cardamom pods, from **Arvinda's Whole Spices**
4-6	**Arvinda's Curry Leaves**
1	medium onion, finely chopped
¼ cup	ground tomatoes
1 ½ tbsp	**Arvinda's Curry Masala**
1 tsp	sea salt OR salt to taste
1 tsp	sugar
1 cup	light cream
¼ cup	ground almonds
1 tbsp	chopped cilantro, to garnish
½ tsp	**Arvinda's Garam Masala**, to garnish

Method of Preparation:

In a pan, heat oil on medium heat. Add cardamom pods and **Arvinda's Curry Leaves** and fry for 1 minute. Add onions and fry until caramelized, approximately 10 minutes.

Add ground tomatoes and fry for 2-3 minutes. Add **Arvinda's Curry Masala**, salt and sugar. Stir and fry masala paste for 2-3 minutes. Add peas and cubed paneer and mix well.

Add cream and ground almonds and stir. Cover and cook for 10 minutes or until the sauce has thickened. Add half a cup of water. Simmer for another 8-10 minutes. This dish should have a thick creamy sauce.

Garnish with cilantro and **Arvinda's Garam Masala**. Serve with Indian flatbreads and rice.

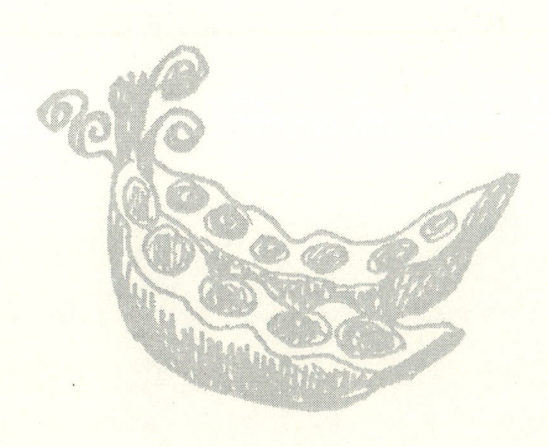

Arvinda and Preena Chauhan

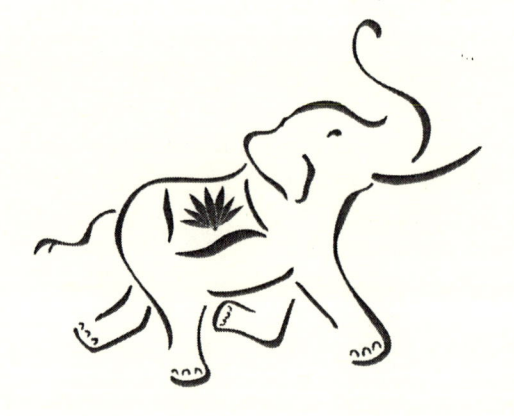

LENTILS & BEANS

India harvests over 60 varieties of lentils and beans. Pulses are an excellent source of protein, minerals, vitamins, dietary fibre and complex carbohydrates, providing nourishment for millions of vegetarians in India. Most Indian meals are served with some kind of lentil or bean dish served with a starch—either rice or flatbread—alongside raita or chutney and a vegetable curry to complete an Indian meal. Lentils can be used to create endless delicious appetizers and desserts as well.

Arvinda's

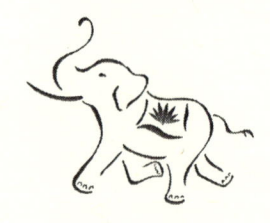

BLACK-EYED BEAN CURRY with SPINACH

This bean dish is healthy with a daily dose of spinach greens.

Ingredients:

1 cup	dried black-eyed beans OR 1 can cooked black-eyed beans
4 cups	water
1 tbsp	oil
1	medium onion, finely chopped
1	medium fresh tomato, chopped
1 ½ tbsp	**Arvinda's Curry Masala**
1 tsp	sea salt
½	bunch fresh spinach, finely chopped
I tbsp	cilantro, to garnish

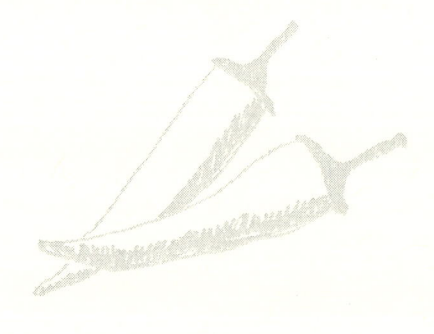

Method of Preparation:

In a large bowl, rinse beans in two to three changes of water. Cover with water and soak overnight.

Wash and drain beans and add to a pot. Add 4 cups of water and boil for 10 minutes. Reduce heat to low and simmer. Keep pan partially covered until beans are tender and cooked. Be sure there is enough water in the pot.

In a separate pan, heat oil on medium high heat. Add onions and cook until soft and golden brown.

Add tomatoes and fry for one minute. Add **Arvinda's Curry Masala** and sea salt. Mix well. Add chopped spinach and cook for 5 minutes.

Stir in cooked black-eyed beans with liquid. Cover and simmer approximately 15 minutes. Add ½ cup of extra water to make a thick curry sauce.

Sprinkle with fresh cilantro to garnish. Serve with chappatis and basmati rice.

Tip:
When out of season, substitute fresh tomato for 1 tablespoon of ground or crushed canned tomatoes.

Arvinda's

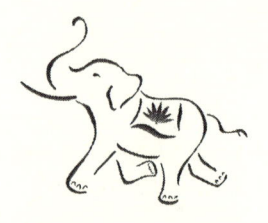

CHANNA DAL with ZUCCHINI
Split Chick Peas with Zucchini

In this dish, an Indian squash called Lauki is traditionally used. Favour local produce and substitute with zucchini which is similar in texture.

Ingredients:

1 cup	channa dal, soaked for 2-3 hours
1	small zucchini squash OR lauki, cubed
6 cups	water
1 tsp	salt
2 tsp	oil
¼ tsp	black mustard seeds
1 tbsp	ground OR crushed tomatoes
1 ½ tbsp	**Arvinda's Curry Masala**
1 tsp	sea salt
1 tsp	sugar
1 tbsp	cilantro, chopped
½ tsp	**Arvinda's Garam Masala**

Method of Preparation:

Wash soaked channa dal in approximately five changes of lukewarm water or until water runs clear.

In a medium pot, simmer channa dal and zucchini in water with salt on medium high heat. Add enough water to cover dal and zucchini. Cover and cook until dal is thoroughly cooked.

In a separate pan, heat oil on medium high heat. Add mustard seeds. Cover pan with a lid and allow mustard seeds to pop. Take care spices do not burn.

Add ground tomatoes, **Arvinda's Curry Masala,** sea salt to taste and sugar. Mix well and fry masala paste for 5 minutes.

Add cooked channa dal and cooked zucchini squash with liquid. Combine with masala paste. Simmer for a few minutes until dal has thickened.

Garnish with cilantro and a sprinkle of **Arvinda's Garam Masala.** Serve with chappatis and basmati rice.

Tip:
To save time, this Channa Dal can be cooked in a pressure cooker in only 5 minutes!

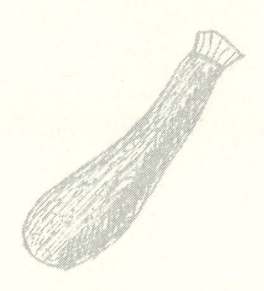

Arvinda's

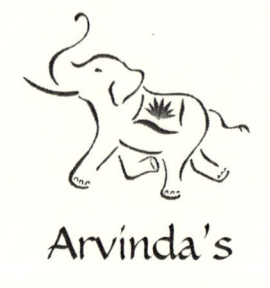

MASOOR DAL
Red Lentil Curry

Ingredients:

1 cup	red split lentils
4 cup	water; add more if necessary
1 tbsp	ghee OR butter
1	small onion, peeled and finely chopped
1 tbsp	**Arvinda's Curry Masala**
1 tsp	salt OR salt to taste
1 tbsp	cilantro, finely chopped
½ tsp	**Arvinda's Garam Masala**, to garnish

Method of Preparation:

Wash lentils in five changes of water until water runs clear. In a medium pot, add enough water to cover lentils and salt. Cover with a lid and simmer on medium heat for 10-15 minutes until lentils are thoroughly cooked.

In a separate pan, melt ghee or butter on medium high heat. Add onions and fry until softened.

Add **Arvinda's Curry Masala** and salt to taste, if necessary. Fry masala until all the spices have blended.

Add cooked lentils to spice mixture. Cover and simmer until lentils thicken.

To serve, garnish with chopped cilantro and a sprinkle of **Arvinda's Garam Masala**. Serve hot with chappatis and rice.

Tip:
This is the ultimate comfort food, perfect for a cold, winter's day!

Arvinda's

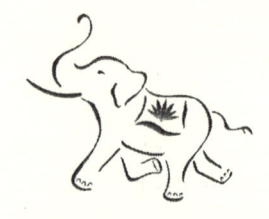

CURRIED CARROT MASOOR DAL SOUP with WHIPPED YOGURT

This is a variation of the previous recipe. More water is added to make the dal a soupy consistency and it is combined with carrots to add natural sweetness.

Ingredients:

2	carrots, cut into small pieces
1 cup	red split lentils
3 cups	water (add more if necessary)
1 tsp	salt
1 tbsp	ghee OR butter
1	medium onion, peeled and finely chopped
1 tbsp	**Arvinda's Curry Masala**
½ cup	2% yogurt
1 tbsp	cilantro, finely chopped, to garnish
½ tsp	**Arvinda's Garam Masala**, to garnish

Method of Preparation:

In a small pot, add carrots and cover with water. Bring to a boil for 10-15 minutes or until carrots are soft.

In a bowl, wash lentils in 4-5 changes of water, until water is clear. Drain.

In a separate medium pot, add lentils, 3 cups of water and salt. Cover and simmer gently for 10-15 minutes until lentils are thoroughly cooked. Set aside.

In a pan, fry onions in ghee until softened. Add **Arvinda's Curry Masala**. Fry until the masala has blended in. Add cooked lentils and cooked carrots. Puree together using a hand blender. Cover and simmer for 10 minutes. Add extra water to thin out soup if necessary.

In a small bowl, whisk yogurt until smooth.

Pour into soup bowls. Garnish with cilantro, whipped yogurt and **Arvinda's Garam Masala**.

Tip:
Serve this soup with pappadum wafers as a garnish. They are available in different flavours from the Indian grocery store.

Arvinda's

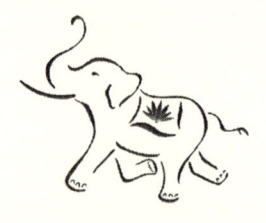

SPROUTED MOONG BEANS

This is a very popular vegetarian dish, which goes well with flatbread, raita and Indian pickles.

Ingredients:

1 cup	whole moong beans, soaked overnight
1 tbsp	oil
2 tbsp	**Arvinda's Curry Masala**
1 tsp	salt OR salt to taste

Method of Preparation:

In a medium bowl, soak whole moong beans in water for 2-3 hours. Wash again in 2-3 changes of water and drain moong beans.

Cover with moist paper towel or damp cheesecloth and leave in a warm place for 2 days, making sure paper towel or cheesecloth is moist at all times. This will allow moong beans to sprout.

Wash and drain sprouted moong beans.

In a pan, heat oil on medium heat. Add moong beans, **Arvinda's Curry Masala** and salt.

Mix well, cover and cook on a low heat until tender. Serve with chappatis or in a pita pocket with tomatoes, lettuce and raita.

Tip:

Other varieties of whole beans can be combined with Moong Beans to make this dish more interesting and to add variation.

Arvinda's

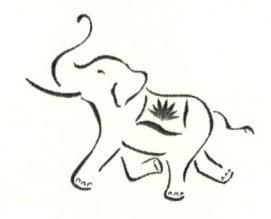

CHANNA MASALA
Whole Chick Pea Curry

Channa masala is typically enjoyed with Naan and Basmati Pullao. For a good lunch option however, serve this curry in a whole wheat pita pocket with lettuce and tomato slices, topped with Cucumber Raita. Perfect for the kids too!

Ingredients:

2 cups	chick peas, canned
3 tbsp	oil
2 -3 each	cardamom pods, cloves, cinnamon bark and star anise from **Arvinda's Whole Spices**
4-6	**Arvinda's Curry Leaves**
1	large onion, finely chopped
2 tbsp	ground tomatoes
1 ½ tbsp	**Arvinda's Curry Masala**
1 tsp	sugar
½ tsp	tamarind paste OR 1 tsp. lemon juice
½ cup	water
1 tsp	sea salt OR salt to taste
2 tbsp	chopped cilantro, to garnish
½ tsp	**Arvinda's Garam Masala**, to garnish

Method of Preparation:

Rinse chick peas and drain. Set aside.

In a medium pan, heat oil on medium high heat. Add **Arvinda's Whole Spices** {cardamom pods, cloves, cinnamon bark and star anise}. Fry until spices sizzle taking care not to burn the spices. Add **Arvinda's Curry Leaves** to hot oil and fry for one more minute.

Add onions and cook until caramelized for approximately 10-15 minutes. Stir in ground tomatoes and cook for one minute. Add **Arvinda's Curry Masala**, sugar and tamarind paste and mix together to make a masala paste. Cook masala for 5 minutes.

Stir in chick peas and add water to make a thick sauce. Add salt to taste. Cover and simmer for 10 minutes.

Garnish with cilantro and **Arvinda's Garam Masala**. Serve with basmati rice and a side salad to make a healthy, well-balanced meal.

Tip:

Try using dried chick peas for this recipe. Soak dried chick peas in water overnight and cook in a pressure cooker for 10 minutes. The taste and texture is lovely — firm with an earthy quality.

Arvinda and Preena Chauhan

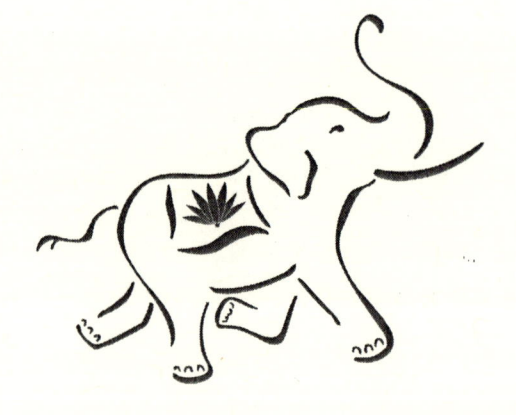

NON-VEGETARIAN CURRIES

Various conquerors journeyed to India over the centuries, heavily influencing its cuisine. North India's cooking reflects more non-vegetarian dishes including Tandoori Chicken, Kebabs and cream-based curry sauces with saffron and nuts. Goa, influenced by the Portuguese, incorporated ingredients native to Europe into curries, such as wine and vinegar in Vindaloo and Madras Curry. Fish dishes are popular in India's coastal regions, specifically the southern province, Kerela. These regional non-vegetarian specialties offer the palate variety and a diversity of flavours.

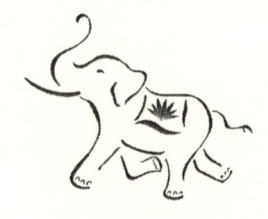

Arvinda's

CLASSIC CHICKEN CURRY
Tomato and Onion-Based Curry with Chicken

Classic chicken curry is a popular and aromatic dish with the use of whole spices. Make it one day ahead so the sauce matures and intensifies.

Ingredients:

4	chicken breasts, cut into pieces
2 tbsp	oil, ghee OR butter
3 each	cardamom pods, cloves, black peppercorns, cinnamon bark and star anise, from **Arvinda's Whole Spices**
1	large onion, peeled and finely chopped
¼ cup	ground OR crushed canned tomatoes
2 tbsp	**Arvinda's Curry Masala**
1 tsp	salt OR salt to taste
½ tsp	nutmeg, freshly grated (optional)
1 cup	water
1 tbsp	cilantro, to garnish
1 tsp	**Arvinda's Garam Masala**, to garnish

Method of Preparation:

In a pan, heat oil or ghee on medium high heat. Add spices from **Arvinda's Whole Spices** {cardamom pods, cloves, black peppercorns, cinnamon bark and star anise}. Fry spices until slightly brown and until they sizzle. Be sure not to burn spices.

Add onions and fry until caramelized. This usually takes 10-15 minutes. Add tomatoes and cook for 2-3 minutes. Add **Arvinda's Curry Masala,** salt and stir fry for 2-3 minutes until it turns into a thick masala paste.

Add chicken pieces and mix with masala. Cover and cook chicken on low heat for 10 minutes.

Add freshly grated nutmeg and mix well. Add water to make a thick curry sauce. Cover and cook until chicken pieces are tender.

Serve in a serving dish and garnish with cilantro and a sprinkling of **Arvinda's Garam Masala**. Serve with rice, Indian flatbread and salad.

Tip:
To make this dish more flavourful use chicken pieces with the bone in.

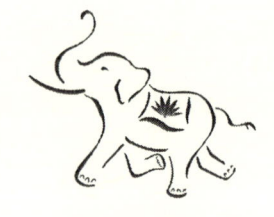

Arvinda's

CURRIED FISH
Fish Pieces in an Aromatic Curry Sauce

Ingredients:

2	white fish fillets, cut into pieces
2 tbsp	oil
2 tbsp	chick pea flour
¼ cup	canned tomatoes, ground or crushed
1 tbsp	**Arvinda's Curry Masala**
1 tsp	salt OR salt to taste
1 cup	water, add more if required
1 tbsp	cilantro, finely chopped
½ tsp	**Arvinda's Garam Masala**

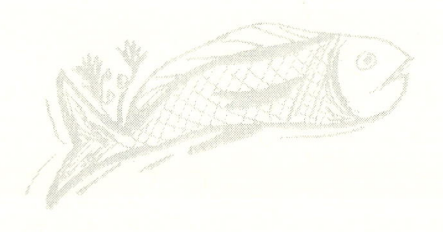

Method of Preparation:

In a medium pan, heat oil on medium high heat. Add chick pea flour and fry until golden brown in colour.

Add ground tomatoes, salt and **Arvinda's Curry Masala**. Fry until masala is blended into a thick paste.

Add water. Whisk or mix well and cook until sauce has thickened.

Add fish pieces and coat well with the sauce. Cook further for about 10 minutes or until fish is cooked.

Garnish with cilantro and a sprinkle of **Arvinda's Garam Masala**. Serve hot with plain boiled rice and a side salad.

Tip:

For this recipe the best fish to use is fillet of tilapia or Haddock, cut into small pieces.

Arvinda's

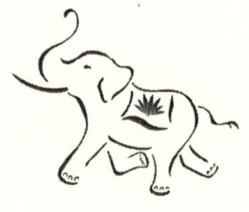

MASALA CHOPS

This is a dry meat dish best served with a salad and a flatbread.

Ingredients:

1 lb	pork OR lamb chops
1 ½ tbsp	**Arvinda's Curry Masala**
½ tsp	salt
2 tbsp	oil
6	lemon wedges
1 tbsp	cilantro, chopped to garnish

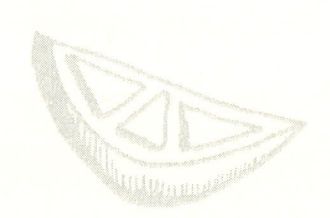

Method of Preparation:

Place chops in a bowl and add **Arvinda's Curry Masala** and salt. Mix spices well into the chops. Marinate for 5-6 hours or overnight in the refrigerator covered.

In a skillet or frying pan, heat oil on medium heat.

Arrange chops in a frying pan and fry for 10-15 minutes each side on low heat until tender and brown. Can also be cooked on the barbecue, basted with oil.

Garnish with cilantro and lemon wedges. Serve with mixed green salad.

Tip:

Add peeled potatoes cut into quarters to the pan and cook with Masala Chops.

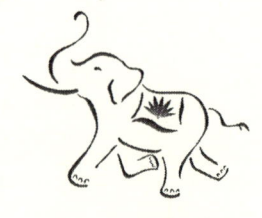

Arvinda's

MADRAS CURRY
Sweet & Sour South Indian-Style Curry

Ingredients

1 lb	chicken OR lamb, cut into small cubes
2 tbsp	**Arvinda's Madras Masala**
1 tbsp	vinegar
2 tbsp	oil OR ghee
1	large onion, finely chopped
¼ cup	ground tomatoes, canned
1 tsp	sugar
½ tsp	tamarind paste
1 cup	water
1 tsp	sea salt OR salt to taste
1 tbsp	chopped cilantro, to garnish
½ tsp	**Arvinda's Garam Masala,** to garnish

Method of Preparation:

In a small bowl combine **Arvinda's Madras Masala** and vinegar together. Mix well to make a smooth paste. Set aside.

In a large pot, heat oil or ghee on medium-high and cook onions until golden brown and caramelized, approximately 10-15 minutes. Add ground tomatoes and fry for 2-3 minutes.

Reduce temperature to medium-low. Add **Arvinda's Madras Masala** with vinegar mixture, salt and mix well. Cook for 2-3 minutes. Add cubed chicken or lamb, stirring until meat is well coated with masala.

Add sugar and tamarind paste and mix well. Add water, cover and simmer on low heat until meat is tender and cooked (15-20 minutes), stirring occasionally.

Transfer to a serving dish and garnish with cilantro and **Arvinda's Garam Masala**.

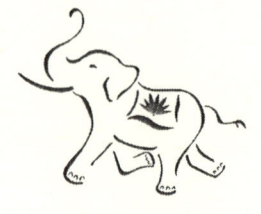

Arvinda's

BOILED EGG CURRY

This is a great curry in a hurry! It is quick, easy to prepare and delicious. Serve with plain boiled rice or Indian flat bread.

Ingredients:

4	hard-boiled eggs, shelled and cut into halves
2 tbsp	oil
3 tbsp	chick pea flour
¼ cup	tomatoes, ground OR crushed, canned
1 ½ tbsp	**Arvinda's Curry Masala**
1 tsp	salt
1 cup	water, add more if required
1 tbsp	cilantro, finely chopped
½ tsp	**Arvinda's Garam Masala**

Method of Preparation:

In a medium non-stick or heavy bottom pan, heat oil on medium heat. Fry chick pea flour in oil until golden brown.

Add ground tomatoes, **Arvinda's Curry Masala** and salt. Fry until all the masala has blended to make a thick paste.

Add water, mix and cook until sauce has thickened.

Add cooked hard-boiled egg halves and coat with sauce. Cook further for about 2-3 minutes.

Serve hot in a serving dish and garnish with cilantro and **Arvinda's Garam Masala**.

Tip:

Plain boiled or steamed rice goes best with this curry because this is a spicy dish.

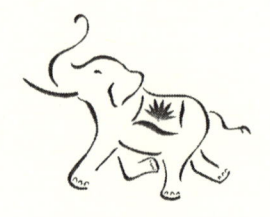

Arvinda's

SHEIKH KEBABS with VEGETABLES

These kebabs can be served with Raita or chutney. Use the meat mixture to make Indian-style burgers or meatballs for a variation.

Ingredients:

1 lb	lean ground lamb, chicken OR turkey meat
1	medium onion, finely chopped
1	whole green chili, finely chopped (optional)
2 tbsp	cilantro, finely chopped
1 tbsp	**Arvinda's Curry Masala**
1 tsp	sea salt OR salt to taste
½ tsp	**Arvinda's Garam Masala**
2 tsp	oil to baste if necessary
12	medium bamboo skewers, soaked in water

Vegetables

1	medium onion, cut into cubes
1	green OR red sweet pepper, cut into cubes
1	firm tomato, cut into cubes

Method of Preparation:

In a bowl mix ground meat, chopped onions, finely chopped chili, cilantro, **Arvinda's Curry Masala**, **Arvinda's Garam Masala** and salt using your hands or a fork. Cover and let mixture stand 10-15 minutes in refrigerator.

Preheat oven to 350F.

Take small lump of meat mixture and form into an oval-shaped kebab and thread onto a bamboo skewer. Add cut onions, peppers and/or tomato on the end of the skewer. Continue with remaining meat mixture and vegetables.

Arrange kebabs on a baking tray and bake in oven until meat is lightly brown for approximately 7 to 10 minutes. Brush with a little oil and flip skewers over and cook for another 4 to 5 minutes.

Serve on bed of lettuce with Green Coriander & Mint Chutney or Cool Cucumber Raita. Serve with a salad, Naan or pita bread.

Tip:

For a summertime variation, use this recipe to make spicy burgers. Form kebab mixture into patties and cook on the barbeque. Serve with Cool Cucumber Raita on a bun with a tomato slice, red onion ring and lettuce.

Arvinda's

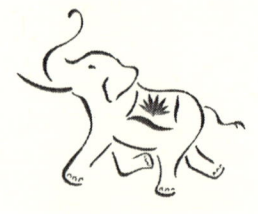

CHICKEN TIKKA

This North Indian dish is very popular as a starter or main course. Substitute paneer or tofu for a vegetarian alternative.

Ingredients:

Marinade:

1 lb	boneless chicken breasts, cubed
¼ cup	plain yogurt
1 tbsp	**Arvinda's Tikka Masala**
1 tsp	lemon juice
2½ tbsp	oil
2	large onions, thinly sliced
½	**each** bell peppers (red, green and yellow), cubed
1 tbsp	**Arvinda's Curry Masala**
1 tsp	salt OR salt to taste
½ tsp	**Arvinda's Garam Masala,** to garnish
2 tbsp	cilantro, finely chopped, to garnish
½	red onion, cut into rounds, to garnish

Method of Preparation:

For this dish the chicken should be marinated overnight or for at least for 3-4 hours.

In a medium bowl add yogurt, **Arvinda's Tikka Masala** and lemon juice. Add chicken cubes and mix well, coating chicken thoroughly. Cover and refrigerate.

In a pan, heat oil on medium-high heat. Add onions and cook until slightly brown. Add **Arvinda's Curry Masala** and salt and mix.

Add marinated chicken and stir in with onions. Cook chicken on low heat until tender. Add additional salt to taste and bell peppers. Mix well and cook further for 5-10 minutes.

Transfer to a serving platter. Garnish with **Arvinda's Garam Masala**, cilantro and red onion rounds. Serve on a bed of basmati rice.

Tip:
Works well on the barbeque!

Arvinda's

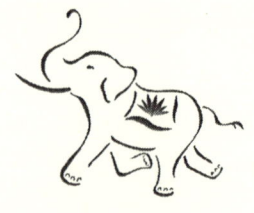

TANDOORI CHICKEN

Ingredients:

3 lbs.	chicken pieces (8-10 legs, thighs OR breasts)
	oil for basting

Marinade:

½ cup	firm plain yogurt
2 tbsp	**Arvinda's Tandoori Masala** OR to taste
1 tbsp	lemon juice
1 tsp	salt OR salt to taste
½ tsp	red food colouring (optional)
1 tbsp	chopped cilantro, to garnish
½ tsp	**Arvinda's Garam Masala,** to garnish

Method of Preparation:

In a large bowl, combine marinade ingredients. Set aside some marinade for basting if cooking on the barbeque. Add chicken pieces and coat evenly. Cover bowl, refrigerate and marinate overnight.

Cook on the barbeque and baste as needed.

Garnish with cilantro and **Arvinda's Garam Masala**.

Option: Place marinated chicken on a foil-lined baking tray and bake in the center of a pre-heated oven at 375F, turning over to achieve even baking. Brush with a little oil and bake (about 15-20 minutes) or until chicken is cooked and slightly brown.

Arvinda and Preena Chauhan

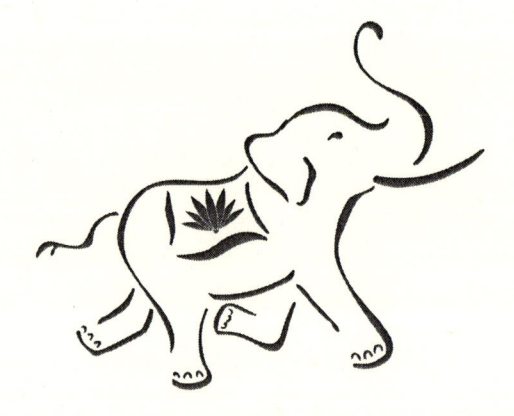

RICE

An Indian meal is incomplete without a serving of rice. Basmati rice is the preferred rice in Indian cuisine and is reserved for the more elaborate North Indian dishes such as Biryani and Pullao. Grown in the northern Indian states, basmati rice is known for its unique aromatic fragrance. Rice nicely compliments both vegetarian and non-vegetarian curries.

Arvinda's

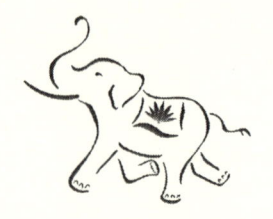

VEGETABLE JEWELLED PULLAO
Mixed Vegetable Rice

This is a beautiful rice dish that adds elegance to any table.

Ingredients:

1 cup	basmati rice, washed
2 tsp	ghee OR oil
2 each	cloves, cardamom, cinnamon sticks, peppercorn and star anise from **Arvinda's Whole Spices**
½ cup	mixed vegetables (frozen peas, carrots & corn)
½ tsp	salt OR salt to taste
1 ½ cup	water, add more if necessary
5	strands of saffron dissolved in 2 tablespoons of milk OR water
1 tbsp	cilantro, finely chopped
½ tsp	**Arvinda's Garam Masala**

Method of Preparation:

In a bowl, wash rice in several changes of warm water until it runs clean. Soak rice in warm water for 10-15 minutes. Drain and set aside.

Heat ghee or oil in a pan on medium heat. Add cloves, cardamom pods, cinnamon sticks, peppercorn and star anise until they sizzle and slightly brown.

Add vegetables and cook for a few minutes. Add strained rice and salt. Gently fold rice making sure it gets evenly coated with ghee, butter or oil.

Add water and bring to a boil. Cover and cook until the water is completely absorbed by the rice. To test if the rice is cooked, mush a grain of rice between the thumb and index finger. If not, sprinkle a little water in the pan, cover and cook further for 2-3 minutes.

In a small bowl, mix saffron with a little water. Let sit for 2 minutes. Fold in saffron with rice. Cover and cook further for few more minutes.

Transfer into serving dish and garnish with **Arvinda's Garam Masala** and cilantro.

Arvinda's

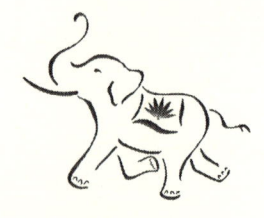

CURRIED RICE
Fine Basmati Rice with Curry Masala

Curried rice is not traditional in India, but the flavours of the spices—chili, coriander, cumin, garlic—add a beautiful complexity to the rice. Turmeric adds colour making this rice dish different from other pullao dishes. Serve with both traditional Indian curries or with non-Indian cuisine as a side.

Ingredients:

1 cup	basmati, parboiled OR long grain rice, washed
2 tsp	ghee OR oil
1 tsp	cumin seeds
2 tbsp	**Arvinda's Curry Masala**
½ tsp	salt OR salt to taste
1 ½ cup	water, add more if necessary
1 tbsp	cilantro, finely chopped (optional)
½ tsp	**Arvinda's Garam Masala**

Method of Preparation:

In a bowl, wash rice in several changes of warm water until it runs clean. Soak rice in warm water for 10-15 minutes. Drain and set aside.

Heat ghee or oil in a pan on medium heat. Add cumin seeds to oil and fry for one minute or until they are golden brown. Add **Arvinda's Curry Masala** and fry for a couple of minutes.

Add strained rice and salt. Gently fold rice making sure rice is evenly coated with ghee, butter or oil.

Add water and bring to a boil. Cover and cook until the water is completely absorbed by the rice. To test if the rice is cooked, mush a grain of rice between the thumb and index finger. If not, sprinkle a little water in the pan, cover and cook further for 2-3 minutes.

Transfer into serving dish and garnish with **Arvinda's Garam Masala** and cilantro.

Arvinda and Preena Chauhan

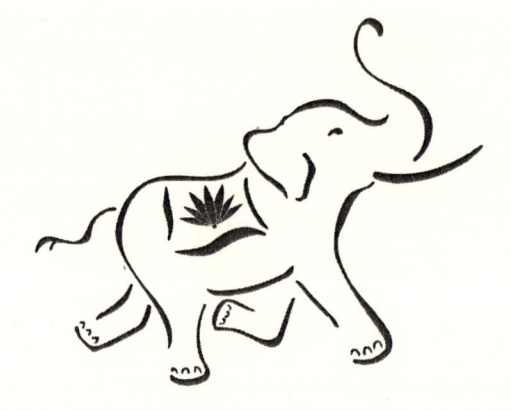

DESSERTS & SWEET BEVERAGES

Indian sweets and desserts are eaten in India for all occasions. There is no auspicious occasion without the presence of Indian sweets especially during Diwali—India's 'Festival of Lights'. Sweets are made from almonds, pistachios, cashews, saffron, milk powder, semolina, cardamom and nutmeg. Often, dessert is served with the main meal, rather than a separate course at the end of a meal.

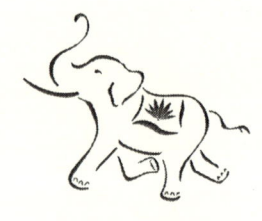

Arvinda's

MASALA CHAI
Spiced Black Tea with Milk & Sugar

Masala Chai is a fragrant spiced tea that is consumed in India at all times of the day. Chai is great on a cold winter's day or even when fighting a bad cold as the spices soothe and provide comfort to the throat. Chai is also decadent enough to be served as a dessert beverage after a meal.

Ingredients:

3 cups	cold water
1 cup	2 % milk
1 tbsp	**Arvinda's Organic Black Loose Tea** OR 2 black tea bags (Orange Pekoe)
1 tsp	**Arvinda's Chai Masala**
½ tsp	fresh ginger, grated (optional)
	sugar to taste

Method of Preparation:

In a medium pot bring cold filtered water to a boil. Add **Arvinda's Organic Black Loose Tea** (or tea bags) and **Arvinda's Chai Masala** and further boil for 3 more minutes.

Add milk and grated ginger (optional).

Boil all the ingredients until tea becomes a caramel colour. Strain in tea pot or tea cups. Serve hot.

Sweeten with sugar or any other sweetener of your choice (raw cane sugar or honey). Enjoy!

Serves 2-4.

Tip:
Add extra fragrance to your Chai by adding pieces of lemongrass to your pot while boiling. Use soy milk or rice milk as a dairy substitute.

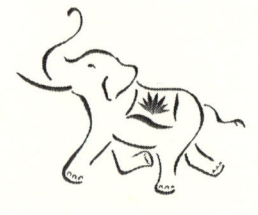

Arvinda's

CHAI VANILLA ICE CREAM with COCONUT & CRANBERRIES

Serve this ice cream as a side to seasonal fruit at the end of an Indian meal.

Ingredients:

3 cups	'real' dairy vanilla ice cream
2 tsp	**Arvinda's Chai Masala**
¼ cup	dried cranberries
2 tbsp	dried unsweetened coconut

Method of Preparation:

Remove ice cream from freezer and allow to sit at room temperature for 5 minutes allowing it to slightly soften.

In a large bowl, combine softened ice cream with **Arvinda's Chai Masala**, dried cranberries and coconut. Mix well.

Transfer into a container and refreeze. Serve with seasonal fruit.

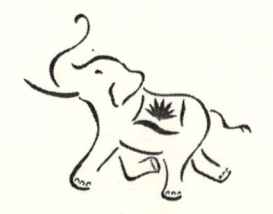

Arvinda's

CRUNCHY CHAI SPICE ALMOND CHOCOLATE & CHERRY BISCOTTI

These biscotti have no butter in them making them crunchy – perfect for dunking in a warm, steamy cup of Masala Chai.

Ingredients:

2	large eggs
¾ cup	sugar
1 tsp	baking powder
2 tsp	pure vanilla extract
2 tsp	**Arvinda's Chai Masala**
1 ½ cup	all-purpose flour
½ cup	dried cherries, coarsely chopped
½ cup	almonds, coarsely chopped
½ cup	dark chocolate, coarsely chopped

Method of Preparation:

Peheat oven to 350F. In a mixing bowl, combine eggs and sugar with an electric mixer. Add baking powder, vanilla and **Arvinda's Chai Masala.**

Add flour and mix well. Fold in dried cherries, almonds and dark chocolate. Form into two logs and place on a baking sheet. Bake for 20 minutes. Cool and slice with serrated knife. Place on baking tray and bake for another 15 minutes.

Arvinda's

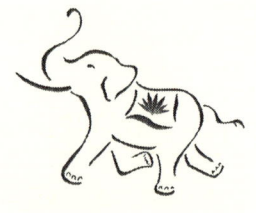

CHAI GINGER RHUBARB APPLES with SEASONAL BERRY COMPOTE

Ingredients:

4	organic apples, peeled, cored, sliced
2	organic rhubarb stems, sliced in small pieces
1 tbsp	ghee OR butter
2 tbsp	brown sugar
1 tsp	**Arvinda's Chai Masala**
½ tsp	ground ginger

Berry compote:

1 cup	water
½ cup	granulated sugar
2 each	**Arvinda's Whole Spices** (excluding black peppercorns)
1 cup	fresh seasonal red fruit (strawberries, sliced OR raspberries)
8	fresh mint leaves, to garnish

Method of Preparation:

Stewed rhubarb and apples: In a pan, melt ghee or butter on medium heat. Add brown sugar and stir with butter. Add rhubarb coating evenly with brown sugar. Cook on medium-low heat until for 10 minutes. Add apples and combine with rhubarb. Cook for another 10 minutes or until softened.

Mix in **Arvinda's Chai Masala** and ground ginger.

Berry compote: In a small saucepan boil water. Add sugar. Simmer on medium and stir to dissolve sugar. Add **Arvinda's Whole Spices**, strawberries or raspberries. Continue to simmer until reduces into a syrup.

Plate apples on dessert plates, garnished with berry compote (remove whole spices when plating dessert) and mint leaves. Serve with Vanilla Chai Spiced Ice Cream on the side.

Serves 6.

Tip:
Try this recipe using whatever soft fruits are in season. In the summer, peaches work wonderful in this dessert.

Arvinda and Preena Chauhan

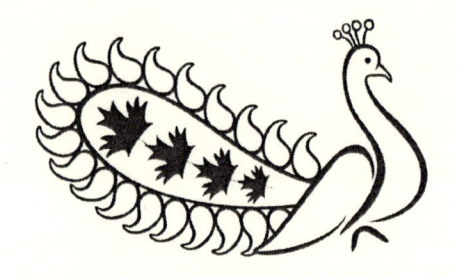

PART 3

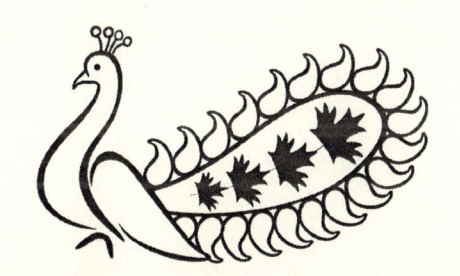

HEALTHY GOURMET INDIAN COOKING recipes

This section features basic and staple recipes essential for any complete Indian meal. All recipes use individual spices.

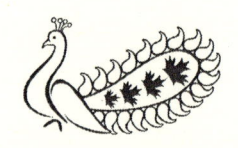

ALOO WADAS
Potato & Cilantro Balls in Chick Pea Batter

Aloo Wadas are a typical Indian deep fried appetizer that can be served hot or cold, making them perfect for a picnic or long journey. Serve with Green Coriander & Mint Chutney.

Ingredients:

Batter
2 cups	chick pea flour
¼ tsp	chili powder
¼ tsp	salt or salt to taste
¼ tsp	baking soda
½ cup	water OR enough water to make thick batter

Filling
5	large potatoes, peeled, boiled and mashed
2 tbsp	cilantro, finely chopped
2 tbsp	raisins
½ tsp	fresh lemon juice
½ tsp	salt OR salt to taste
½ tsp	**Arvinda's Garam Masala**
¼ tsp	chili powder
	oil for deep frying

Method of Preparation:

Batter: In a medium bowl sift chick pea flour.

Add chili powder, salt and baking powder. Add enough water to make a thick smooth batter. If batter is too thin add extra sifted chick pea flour to thicken it up. Batter should be of a thick consistency. Set aside to rest.

Filling: In a large bowl, mix mashed potatoes with the rest of the filling ingredients. Mix well.

Take a small lump of the filling mixture the size of a walnut and form a smooth ball. Continue to mold the remaining mixture the same way.

In a pan, wok or kadhai, heat oil for deep frying on medium temperature.

Dip potato wadas (balls) in chick pea flour batter, coating well. Slide each ball into the oil carefully. Fry until golden brown. Remove from the oil and drain on a paper towel.

Tip:
Aloo wadas can be prepared and fried ahead of time, and reheated in the oven before serving.

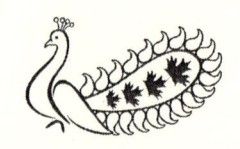

MIXED VEGETABLE PAKORAS
Mixed Vegetable Chick Pea Fritters

Ingredients:

Batter mixture

2 cup	chick pea (besan OR gram) flour
½ tsp	ajwan seeds (optional)
½ tsp	salt OR salt to taste
¼ tsp	baking powder OR soda
¼ tsp	chili powder
¼ cup	water

Vegetables

2	small potatoes, peeled, finely chopped
1	small zucchini, finely chopped
1	small onion, finely chopped
2	green pepper, seeded, finely chopped
1	small ripe banana, finely chopped (optional)
¼ cup	cilantro, finely chopped
2 cup	light cooking oil for deep frying

Method of Preparation:

Batter: In a mixing bowl, combine chick pea flour, ajwan seeds, salt, baking soda and chili powder. Add water, mix and combine to make a thick batter.

Add chopped vegetables. Mix well and allow to stand for 5 minutes.

In a kadhai or wok, heat oil on medium heat for deep-frying.

Take a teaspoon of mixture and carefully drop in oil. Fry a few at a time. Fry on all sides until golden brown.

Drain well on a paper towel. Serve hot or cold with chutneys.

Tip:

This appetizer is a good option for anyone who has a gluten allergy as it contains no wheat. If you don't have a spicy chutney on hand, serve these pakoras with ketchup.

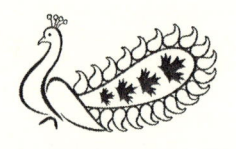

GREEN CILANTRO & MINT CHUTNEY

This chutney's freshness makes it a versatile condiment that can be served with almost all Indian appetizers.

Ingredients:

1 cup	cilantro, finely chopped
½ cup	fresh mint leaves
1 tsp	fresh lemon juice
½ tsp	salt
½ tsp	whole cumin seeds
1	green chili
1	small apple, peeled and cubed
1	medium fresh tomato, cubed
1	garlic clove

Method of Preparation:

In a blender, mix all ingredients together.

Blend on medium speed until mixture is smooth. Makes ¾ cup (125 mL).

Tip:

For added hotness, add one or two extra chilies. This fresh chutney will last 5 days in the refrigerator. Combine this chutney with yogurt for a variation.

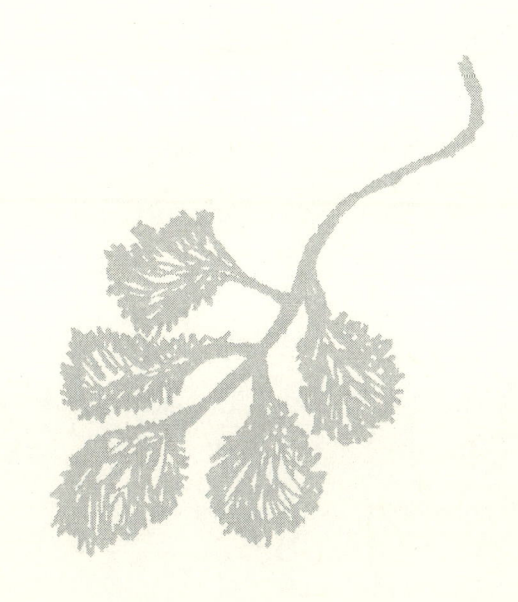

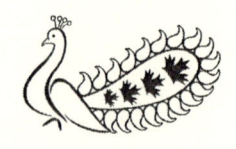

SWEET & SOUR TAMARIND DATE CHUTNEY

Serve with Indian snacks.

Ingredients:

1 cup	pitted dates
1 tbsp	tamarind paste
½ tsp	salt OR salt to taste
½ tsp	**Arvinda's Garam Masala**
¼ tsp	chili powder (add more for hotness)

Method of Preparation:

In a small bowl, wash pitted dates. Cover with warm water and soak overnight.

In a blender, add dates with liquid, tamarind paste, salt, **Arvinda's Garam Masala** and chili powder.

Combine all the ingredients until smooth.

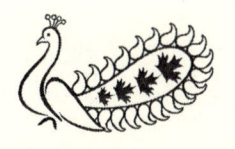

SWEET APPLE CHUTNEY

Serve with a full Indian meal.

Ingredients:

3	organic apples, peeled and grated
¼ cup	sugar
1 tbsp	vinegar
½ tsp	whole cumin seeds
½ tsp	chili powder
½ tsp	salt
3	cinnamon bark, from **Arvinda's Whole Spices**
3	cloves, from **Arvinda's Whole Spices**

Method of Preparation:

In a heavy bottom pot, mix grated apples with the rest of the ingredients on low heat.

Simmer and cook for 45 minutes to an hour or until mixture is soft, dry and dark in colour. All moisture should be absorbed.

Serve with vegetarian curries.

Tip:
Store this preserved chutney in a glass jar in the refrigerator.

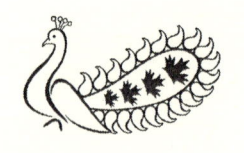

MANGO PICKLES

This pickle is typically served with a vegetarian Indian meal as a side garnish. Serve also with Indian flatbreads.

Ingredients:

2	small firm green mangoes, finely cubed
½ cup	oil, OR enough oil to coat fruit evenly
2 tbsp	mustard seeds, coarsely ground
2 tbsp	fenugreek seeds, coarsely ground
1 tsp	chili powder
½ tsp	salt OR salt to taste

Method of Preparation:

Place chopped mangoes in a small bowl and add all other ingredients. Mix thoroughly. Store pickles in a jar.

Can be refrigerated in a jar for a week or longer if enough oil is added to preserve the fruit. Serve with dals or vegetarian dishes.

Tip:

Julianne carrots and green chilies can be added to this recipe for a variation. Green apples can be substituted for the green mangoes.

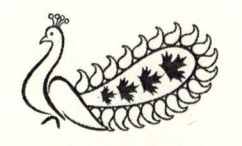

COOL CUCUMBER RAITA
Yogurt with Grated Cucumber

Ingredients:

½	English cucumber, grated finely
1 cup	firm yogurt
½ tsp	cumin seeds, roasted and ground
½ tsp	black mustard seeds, crushed
½ tsp	garlic puree
¼ tsp	salt, OR salt to taste

Garnish
1 tbsp	cilantro, finely chopped
½ tsp	**Arvinda's Garam Masala**
¼ tsp	chili powder

Method of Preparation:

In a medium bowl, combine grated cucumber with yogurt, ground cumin, crushed mustard seeds, garlic puree and salt. Mix well. Chill until serving with the meal.

Garnish before serving with a sprinkle of fresh cilantro, **Arvinda's Garam Masala** and chili powder.

Tip:
Choose non-fat yogurt for a healthier option.

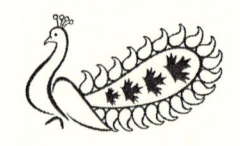

KACHUMBER
Indian Tomato & Cucumber Salad

Typically Indian salad dressings consist of lemon juice, vinegar, sea salt and spices.

Ingredients:

Dressing
1 tbsp	fresh lemon juice
1 tbsp	vinegar
1 tsp	sugar
¼ tsp	chili powder (optional)
½ tsp	**Arvinda's Garam Masala**
½ tsp	sea salt

Vegetables
2	carrots, grated
2	firm tomatoes, finely cubed
2	red onions, finely chopped OR sliced
½	cucumber, finely cubed
¼ cup	fresh cilantro, finely chopped
6	mint leaves, finely chopped

Method of Preparation:

Dressing: In a small bowl, add lemon juice, vinegar, sugar, chili powder, **Arvinda's Garam Masala** and salt. Mix well and set aside.

In a large bowl, combine onions, tomatoes, carrots, cucumber and cilantro. Add dressing and toss well.

Chill in refrigerator and garnish with mint before serving.
Serve as a compliment to any Indian meal.

Tip:

For this recipe, use red wine or balsamic vinegar for added flavour to the dressing. Add some radishes for a variation.

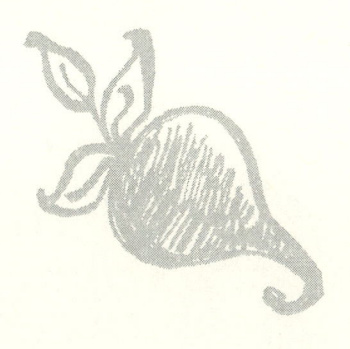

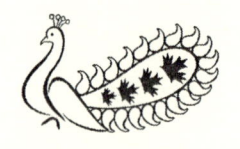

CARROT & CABBAGE SAMBAR
Sweet & Sour Warm Indian-Style Coleslaw

Ingredients:

2 tsp	oil
½ tsp	brown mustard seeds
2	medium carrots, peeled and grated
1	green chilies, sliced (optional)
½	sweet bell pepper, sliced
¼	medium cabbage, finely shredded
1 tsp	sugar
½ tsp	salt OR salt to taste
½ tsp	lemon juice
¼ tsp	turmeric powder

Method of Preparation:

In a wok or kadhai, heat oil on medium to high heat. Fry mustard seeds in oil until they sizzle.

Add carrots, chilies, bell peppers and cabbage. Combine.

Add sugar, salt, lemon juice and turmeric powder.

Mix well and stir fry for a few minutes. Be sure not to overcook vegetables. Serve as a side dish.

Tip:
Mustard seeds expand and pop when added to hot oil, so put a lid on the pan when frying.

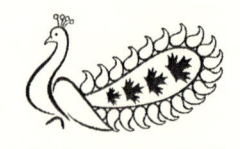

CHAPPATI
Pan-Broiled Round Wheat Indian Flatbread

The world's simplest and healthiest bread, Chappatis are a delicate Indian flatbread that goes with both non-vegetarian and vegetarian curries. This flatbread is an 'everyday' bread cooked daily for most meals in India.

Ingredients:

1 cup	duram flour
1 cup	soft whole wheat flour (chappati flour)
1 tsp	oil
¾ cup	warm water OR as required to make a soft pliable dough

Method of Preparation:

Place flour in a large mixing bowl or dish. Add oil, and using your fingers mix well. Gradually add water and knead. Add enough water to make soft pliable dough. Cover and set aside to rest for 10-15 minutes.

Take a lump of dough of the size of a golf ball. On a lightly floured counter or pastry board, roll one at a time in the shape of a circle relative to the size of a tortilla.

Heat a non-stick frying pan or griddle on high heat. Place a rolled chappati on the griddle and cook for 1-2 minutes on each side until little brown specks appear. At this time, apply pressure to the chappati by pressing with tea cloth. This will allow them to puff up. Cook on both sides.

Make the rest in the same way and stack them in a pile. Add a little butter or ghee to keep chappati soft on one side, however this is optional. Keep them warm, covered in a chappati container or in foil. Serve with vegetarian or non-vegetarian curries.

Tip:

Chappatis can be prepared ahead of time. Wrap in foil and warm them in a 250F heated oven for 10 minutes. Chappatis can be cooked directly on the electric element of the stove (or on the gas stove) by placing them on a cake wire rack. Take care not to burn them.

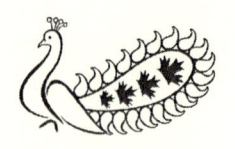

PURI
Deep-Fried Small Round Flatbread

While Chappatis are served fresh daily for all meals, Puris are reserved for special occasions or for guests. They are served best with vegetarian curries.

Ingredients:

1 cup	chappati OR soft whole wheat flour
1 cup	duram flour
¼ cup	semolina (suji)
1 tsp	oil
½ tsp	salt
¾ cup	warm water, OR enough to make a stiff dough
	oil for deep frying

Method of Preparation:

In a large mixing bowl combine flours, salt and oil. Mix well and knead with warm water to make stiff dough. If you add too much water, add more flour. Knead well and allow to stand covered for 5-10 minutes.

Take small lump of dough in the size of golf ball and roll it out into a small circle on an oiled surface.

In a wok, heat oil to medium heat for deep frying. Slide one puri into the oil at a time. Press puri gently with a straining spoon. Turn over and allow the puri to swell. It may need a little pressure to puff up.

Cook for 1-2 minutes until light golden brown on both sides. Fry all the puris and serve hot.

Tip:

To test the temperature of the oil, drop a piece of dough into hot oil. When the dough surfaces immediately the oil is ready. Be sure oil does not fume.

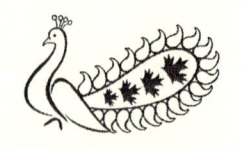

ALOO GOBI
Cauliflower Curry with Potatoes & Peas

This cauliflower curry is the definitive vegetarian dish. Serve with Chappati.

Ingredients:

2 tbsp	oil
½ tsp	brown mustard seeds
½ tsp	cumin seeds
4-6	**Arvinda's Curry Leaves**
2	medium potatoes, peeled and cubed
1 cup	peas
½	small cauliflower, cut into small pieces
2 tsp	ground cumin & coriander powder
1 tsp	salt OR salt to taste
½ tsp	turmeric powder
½ tsp	chili powder
1 tbsp	cilantro, to garnish
½ tsp	**Arvinda's Garam Masala**

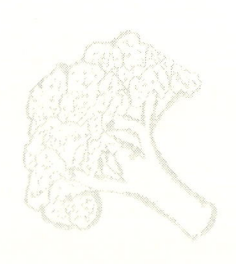

Method of Preparation:

In a pan, heat oil on medium-high temperature. Add mustard and cumin seeds. Cover and wait until they pop. Add **Arvinda's Curry Leaves** and fry for one minute.

Add potatoes, peas and cauliflower. Lower temperature to medium low heat.

Add cumin & coriander powder, salt, turmeric powder and chili powder. Mix well to coat potatoes and cauliflower with oil and spices.

Cover and cook on low heat until potatoes are tender and cooked.

Garnish with cilantro and **Arvinda's Garam Masala**.

Tip:

Make this curry moist by adding ¼ cup of ground tomatoes and 1 cup of water to make thick gravy. Add extra spices if necessary as they will be diluted when extra ingredients are added.

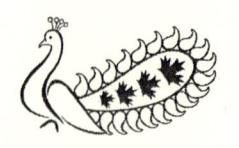

CHANNA DAL WITH ZUCCHINI
Split Chick Peas with Zucchini

Ingredients:

1 cup	channa dal, soaked for 2-3 hours
1	small zucchini, cubed
6 cups	water
1 tsp	salt
2 tsp	oil
¼ tsp	brown mustard seeds
2 tbsp	ground OR crushed tomatoes, canned
1 tsp	cumin & coriander powder
1 tsp	sugar
½ tsp	garlic puree
¼ tsp	chili powder
¼ tsp	turmeric powder
1 tbsp	cilantro, chopped
½ tsp	**Arvinda's Garam Masala**

Method of Preparation:

Wash soaked channa dal in five changes of water, or until water runs clear. Drain.

In a medium pot, add 6 cups of water, salt, channa dal and zucchini. Simmer on medium high heat. Cover and cook until dal is thoroughly cooked.

In a separate pan on medium high heat, add oil and mustard seeds. Cover pan with a lid and fry mustard seeds until they pop.

Add ground tomatoes, cumin & coriander powder, sugar, garlic puree, turmeric powder and chili powder. Fry masala mixture for 3 minutes.

Add cooked channa dal and cooked zucchini with liquid. Mix well. Simmer for 10 minutes until dal has thickened.

Garnish with cilantro and **Arvinda's Garam Masala**. Serve with Chappati or basmati rice.

Tip:
To save time cook the Channa Dal in a pressure cooker, which only takes five minutes to cook!

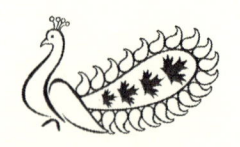

MASOOR DAL
Red Lentil Curry

This lentil curry has a soupy consistency. This is comfort food at its best!

Ingredients:

1 cup	red split lentils
3 cup	water (add more if necessary)
1 tbsp	ghee OR butter
1	small onion, peeled and finely chopped
1 tsp	salt OR salt to taste
2 tsp	cumin & coriander powder
½ tsp	garlic puree
½ tsp	turmeric powder
½ tsp	chili powder
1 tbsp	cilantro, finely chopped, to garnish
½ tsp	**Arvinda's Garam Masala**, to garnish

Method of Preparation:

Wash lentils in five changes of water or until water runs clear. Add to a medium pot with water and salt. Partially cover and simmer on medium heat for 10-15 minutes until lentils are thoroughly cooked.

In a separate pan, melt ghee or butter on medium high heat. Add onions and fry until they become softened.

Add cumin & coriander powder, garlic puree, turmeric powder and chili powder. Fry masala until spices are combined.

Add cooked lentils to spice mixture. Mix, cover and simmer until lentils thicken. This dish should have a soupy consistency.

To serve, garnish with chopped cilantro and **Arvinda's Garam Masala**. Serve hot with Chappati or rice.

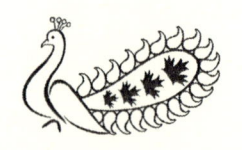

CHANNA MASALA
Whole Chick Pea Curry

This is a popular chick pea curry as it's tasty and makes for a satisfying, healthy meal when served with Chappati. Try serving it in a pita pocket with lettuce, tomatoes and Raita.

Ingredients:

1 cup	dried chick peas, soaked overnight
1 tsp	salt
3 tsp	oil
5-6	**Arvinda's Curry Leaves**
3	cardamom pods, from **Arvinda's Whole Spices**
2	cinnamon, from **Arvinda's Whole Spices**
1	onion, finely chopped
¼ cup	crushed OR ground tomatoes, canned
½ tsp	ginger puree
½ tsp	garlic puree
1 tsp	cumin & coriander powder
1 tsp	sugar
½ tsp	chili powder
½ tsp	tamarind paste
¼ tsp	turmeric powder
1 tbsp	cilantro, finely chopped, to garnish
½ tsp	**Arvinda's Garam Masala**, to garnish

Method of Preparation:

Rinse chick peas and place them in a medium bowl. Cover with water and soak overnight.

Wash and drain chick peas. In a medium pot add chick peas, salt and cover with water. Boil for 10 minutes. Reduce heat and simmer, partially covered for 1 hour until chick peas are tender. Be sure there is enough water in a pot.

In a separate pan, heat oil on medium high heat. Add **Arvinda's Curry Leaves**, cardamom pods and cinnamon sticks and temper in oil until they sizzle.

Add onions and cook until golden brown and caramelized, approximately 10-15 minutes. Add crushed tomatoes and fry for one minute. Add ginger puree, garlic puree, cumin & coriander powder, sugar, tamarind paste, chili powder and turmeric powder. Add salt to taste. Stir and cook masala for 5 minutes.

Stir in cooked chick peas, cover and simmer until they are tender. Add enough water (½ cup) to make a thick sauce.

Garnish with cilantro and **Arvinda's Garam Masala.** Serve with basmati rice and Raita, which serves as a well balanced meal.

Tip:

For this recipe use two small cans of chick peas for convenience. Rinse well before using. Tamarind paste can be substituted for 1 tsp of lemon juice.

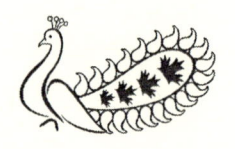

BOILED OR STEAMED RICE

Ingredients:

1 cup	long-grain OR basmati rice
1 ½ cup	water, add an extra ½ cup if necessary
1 tsp	butter OR ghee
½ tsp	salt

Method of Preparation:

In a large bowl, wash rice in five changes of warm water until water runs clear. Set aside for 10-15 minutes and fill bowl with enough warm water to cover rice.

Wash rice again in a couple changes of water. Drain rice through a strainer. On medium heat, add butter or ghee to pan. Add rice and salt. Gently fold rice, so grains are coated with butter or ghee. Add water. Cover and gently bring to boil until the water is absorbed.

Keep on low heat for a few minutes to evaporate any remaining moisture and complete cooking rice. To test if rice is fully cooked, take a grain and mush between you thumb and index finger to test. If it is hard, add a little water and further cook for few more minutes.

Fluff with a fork and serve with Indian curries.

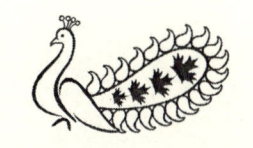

JEERA RICE
Basmati Rice with Whole Cumin Seeds

Ingredients:

1 cup	basmati rice
2 tsp.	oil OR ghee
1 ½ cups	water
½ tsp.	whole cumin seeds
½ tsp.	sea salt
1 tsp.	**Arvinda's Garam Masala**

Method of Preparation:

In a medium bowl, wash rice in 4-5 changes of water and soak in warm water for 10-15 minutes.

Wash again in a few changes of water until water is clear. Handle rice carefully so grains do not break. Drain and set aside.

In a pan, heat ghee or oil on medium heat. Add whole cumin seeds and fry until slightly browned. Add strained rice and salt. Gently fold rice ensuring grains are evenly coated with ghee or oil.

Add water, bring to a boil and cover and cook on low heat until water is completely absorbed. Add a little water if necessary. Cover and cook further for few more minutes.

Garnish with **Arvinda's Garam Masala**. Serve hot with curries.

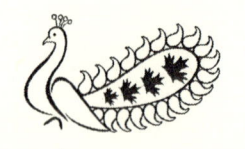

MATTAR RICE
Basmati Rice with Peas

This is a more elaborate rice dish that can be paired with any curry.

Ingredients:

1 cup	basmati rice
1 tbsp	ghee OR oil
½ tsp	whole cumin seeds
½ cup	frozen peas
½ tsp	salt
½ tsp	turmeric powder
1 ½ cup	water, add ¼ cup more, if necessary

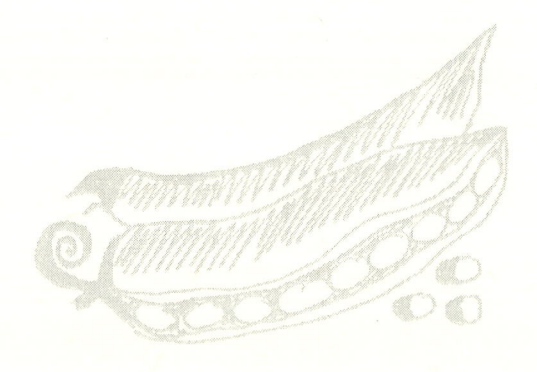

Method of Preparation:

In a medium bowl, wash rice in five changes of lukewarm water until water runs clear. Cover with lukewarm water and soak rice for 10-15 minutes. Strain and set aside.

Heat ghee or oil in a pan on medium heat. Add cumin seeds and fry until they sizzle and slightly brown.

Add strained rice, peas, turmeric powder and salt. Mix well making sure rice is evenly coated with ghee, butter or oil.

Add water, bring to a boil, cover and cook on low heat until water is completely absorbed. Test if rice is cooked by mushing a grain between thumb and a finger. If grains are hard, sprinkle in a little water, cover and cook further for 2-3 minutes.

Transfer into serving dish and serve with curry.

Tip:
When washing basmati rice be sure to wash with care. Basmati grains are fine and delicate and can break easily, which will in turn make your rice mushy.

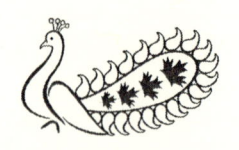

INDIAN-STYLE RICE PUDDING WITH SAFFRON & NUTS

Known as Kheer, this rice pudding is a very popular dessert in North India. It is also an auspicious dessert served during the Indian festivals.

Ingredients:

½ cup	short-grain rice
5 cups	milk
1 can	evaporated milk
5 tbsp	sugar OR sugar to taste
1 tbsp	almonds, finely chopped
1 tbsp	raw pistachio nuts, finely chopped
½ tsp	cardamom seeds, ground
½ tsp	nutmeg, freshly grated
¼ tsp	saffron, soaked in water OR milk

Method of Preparation:

Soak rice in warm water for 10-15 minutes. Wash in three changes of water. Drain rice and put in a large heavy-bottomed pot or a non-stick pot.

Add milk and bring it to a boil. Reduce heat to low heat. Cook until the rice pudding is fairly thick (takes approximately 45 minutes to one hour). Stir occasionally.

Add evaporated milk and sugar and cook further for a few more minutes.

Add saffron and stir. Remove rice pudding from heat and transfer into serving dish. Garnish with chopped almonds and pistachio, ground cardamom and nutmeg.

Tip:
Serve warm or chilled. This rice pudding can also be served as a side to a vegetarian main meal.

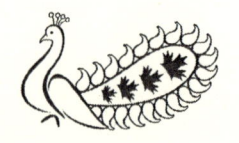

MANGO LASSI
Cool Indian Yogurt Beverage with Mango

Ingredients:

1 cup	plain yogurt
1 cup	light cream, milk OR water
1 cup	mango pulp or puree
¼ cup	sugar OR add more to taste
2 cups	crushed ice
4-6	mint leaves

Method of Preparation:

Blend all the above ingredients except mint leaves in a blender until smooth and creamy.

Serve in a tall glass and garnish with mint leaves.

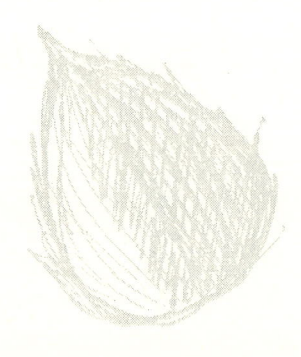

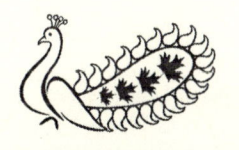

GAJJAR KA HALWA
Carrot & Raisin Halwa (Sweetmeat)

Ingredients:

3 lbs	carrots, peeled and finely grated
1 can	evaporated milk
2 tbsp	ghee OR unsalted butter
1 ½ cups	sugar
¼ cup	raisins
¼ cup	raw cashews, halved
1 tsp	cardamoms seeds, crushed
1 tsp	nutmeg, grated
1 tbsp	almonds, chopped, to garnish
1 tbsp	pistachio nuts, chopped, to garnish

Method of Preparation:

Heat evaporated milk and ghee or butter in a heavy bottom or non-stick pan set on low heat.

Add grated carrots and cook on low heat until they are tender and caramelized. Colour should change from orange to deep red or brown. This takes approximately 1 hour.

Add sugar, raisins and cashews. Continue to cook on low heat for another 30-45 minutes, constantly stirring (otherwise it will stick to the pan). Sprinkle cardamom seeds and grated nutmeg and mix. Serve warm in a serving bowls and garnish with chopped nuts.

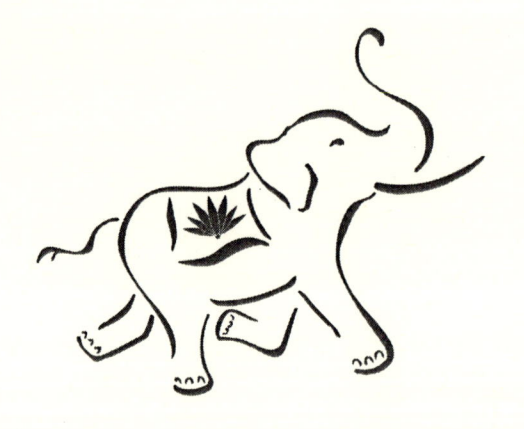

APPENDICES

TABLE OF CONVERSIONS

Metric	Imperial

Oven Temperature

Metric	Imperial
120 °C	250 F
140 °C	275 F
150 °C	300 F
160 °C	325 F
180 °C	350 F
190 °C	375 F
200 °C	400 F
220 °C	425 F
230 °C	450 F
240 °C	475 F
260 °C	500 F

Mass

Metric	Imperial
25 g	1 oz
50 g	2 oz
75 g	3 oz
125 g	4 oz = ¼ lb
150 g	5 oz
175 g	6 oz
250 g	8 oz = ½ lb
300 g	10 oz
375 g	12 oz = ¾ lb
500 g	16 oz = 1 lb
1.0 kg	2 lb
1.5 kg	3 lb
2.0 kg	4 lb

Volume

Metric	Imperial
1 mL	¼ tsp
2 mL	½ tsp
4 mL	¾ tsp
5 mL	1 tsp
15 mL	1 tbsp
30 mL	2 tbsp
45 mL	3 tbsp
50 mL	¼ cup
75 mL	1/3 cup
125 mL	½ cup
150 mL	2/3 cup
175 mL	¾ cup
250 mL	1 cup
1 L	4 cups

ARVINDA'S ARTISANAL SPICE BLENDS

Arvinda's line consists of some of the following products. For information on the full line, please refer to www.arvindas.com. Purchase online at www.hgic.ca/store.htm.

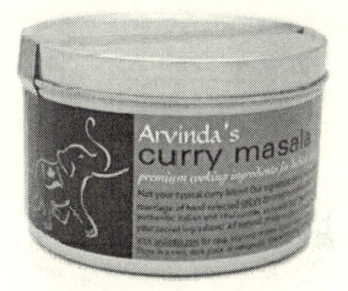

Arvinda's Curry Masala
Not your typical curry blend! Our signature blend is an epicurean marriage of hand selected spices and fresh garlic & ginger used to create endless healthy and delicious Indian and Thai curries. Excellent for grilling marinades. Versatile and ingenious, this is *your* secret ingredient!

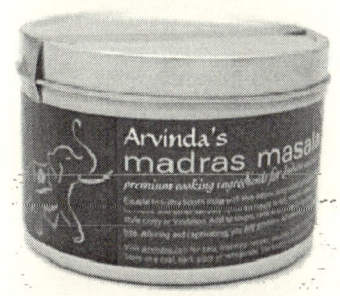

Arvinda's Madras Masala
Escape to sultry South India with this intoxicating blend of black pepper, turmeric and other savoury spices to create rich, mouth-watering Madras style curries or Vindaloo. Add to soups, raita and sauces for an exotic Indian bite. Alluring and captivating, you are smitten.

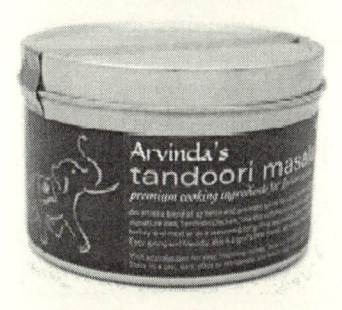

Arvinda's Tandoori Masala
An artistic blend of 17 herbs and aromatic spices to create North India's succulent signature dish, Tandoori Chicken. Use this symphonic blend as a spice rub for roast turkey, meat or grilling vegetables or as a seasoning for salmon and fish. Easy-going and friendly, this is a grill's best friend.

Arvinda's Tikka Masala
Fire up your taste buds with our most dynamite spice blend. Take the fast lane to make a yogurt based marinade for Chicken Tikka or heighten your vegetables to the extreme. Add risk to your ribs and danger to your grilling marinades. Caution: You are playing with fire.

Arvinda's Garam Masala
Worthy of royalty, this delicate spice blend is an opulent combination of premium, hand-selected spices, roasted and ground into a tapestry of luxuriant flavours. Like a touch of gold, add a sprinkle on your favourite Indian curries and rice dishes for a warm, perfumed finish.

INDEX

ALOO WADAS, 20, 110
ALOO GOBI, 54, 128
Arvinda's Products, C
Ajwan seeds, 5
Asafoetida, 5
Belen, 9
BLACK-EYED BEAN CURRY, 64
BOILED EGG CURRY, 86
BOILED OR STEAMED RICE, 136
Cardamom, 5
CARROT & CABBAGE SAMBAR, 38, 122
CHAI GINGER RHUBARB APPLES with SEASONAL BERRY COMPOTE, 106
CHAI VANILLA ICE CREAM with COCONUT & CRANBERRIES, 104
CHAI VANILLA YOGURT with SEASONAL SOFT FRUIT & WALNUTS, 51
CHANNA DAL with ZUCCHINI, 66, 130
CHANNA MASALA, 74, 134
CHAPPATI, 124
Chick pea flour, 5
CHICKEN TIKKA, 90
Chilies, 5
Cinnamon, 6
CLASSIC CHICKEN CURRY, 78
Cloves, 6
Coriander, 6
CRUNCHY CHAI SPICE ALMOND CHOCOLATE & CHERRY BISCOTTI, 105
Cumin Seeds, 6
CURRIED APPLE PRESERVES, 36
CURRIED CARROT, 70
CURRIED FISH, 80
CURRIED MAPLED WALNUTS, 33
CURRIED PUMPKIN APPLE SOUP, 28
CURRIED RICE, 98

Curry Leaves, 6
dabba. See Masala box
Dal, 6
DAL WADAS, 22
Fennel Seeds, 7
Fenugreek Seeds, 7
Food Processor, 9
GAJJAR KA HALWA, 143
Garam Masala, 7
GARAM MASALA OMELETTES, 48
Garlic, 7
Ghee, 7
GHEE, 13
Ghee Container, 9
Ginger, 7
GREEN CILANTRO & MINT CHUTNEY, 114
hing. See Asafoetida
INDIAN-STYLE PANCAKES, 49
INDIAN-STYLE RICE PUDDING WITH SAFFRON & NUTS, 140
Jaggery, 7
JEERA RICE, 137
KACHUMBER, 120
Kadhai, 9
MADRAS CURRY, 84
MADRAS VEGETABLE RAITA, 37
MADRASI FRENCH TOAST, 50
MANGO LASSI, 142
MANGO PICKLES, 118
Masala box, 9
MASALA CHAI, 102
MASALA CHOPS, 82
MASALA PURI, 44
MASOOR DAL, 68, 132
MATTAR PANEER, 60
MATTAR RICE, 138
METHI THEPLA, 42
MIXED VEGETABLE CURRY, 56
MIXED VEGETABLE PAKORAS, 26, 112
Mortar & pestle, 9
Mustard Seeds, 7

Nutmeg, 8
ORGANIC HOMEMADE YOGURT, 14
PANEER, 12
Parat, 9
Pressure Cooker, 10
PURI, 126
Saffron, 8
Saucepan, 10
SEASONED TOFU, 32, 33
SHEIKH KEBABS with VEGETABLES, 88
SPICED POTATO &, 58

SPROUTED MOONG BEANS, 72
SWEET & SOUR TAMARIND, 116
SWEET APPLE CHUTNEY, 117
Tamarind, 8
TANDOORI CHICKEN, 92
Tawa, 10
Thali, 10
TIKKA POTATOES, 30
Turmeric, 8
VEGETABLE JEWELLED PULLAO, 96
WHOLE VEGETABLE PAKORAS, 24